# FOOT SCIENCE

A Selection of Papers from the Proceedings of the
American Orthopaedic Foot Society, Inc., 1974 and 1975

*Edited by*

## JAMES E. BATEMAN, M.D., F.R.C.S.(C.)

Surgeon-in-Chief, Orthopaedic and Arthritic Hospital,
Toronto, Ontario

W. B. SAUNDERS COMPANY • Philadelphia • London • Toronto

W. B. Saunders Company:  West Washington Square
Philadelphia, Pa.  19105

1 St. Anne's Road
Eastbourne, East Sussex BN21 3UN, England

833 Oxford Street
Toronto, M8Z 5T9, Canada

**Library of Congress Cataloging in Publication Data**

American Orthopaedic Foot Society.
  Foot science.

  Includes index.

  1.  Foot—Abnormities and deformities.  2.  Foot—Surgery.  3.  Ankle—Surgery.
I.  Bateman, James Ennis, 1915-    .  II.  Title.  [DNLM:  1.  Foot diseases—Congresses.  2.  Orthopedics—Congresses.  WE880  F687]

RD781.A52  1976     617.5'85     75-14780
ISBN 0-7216-1580-5

Foot Science                                                    ISBN  0-7216-1580-5

Last digit is the print number:     9    8    7    6    5    4    3    2

# Contributors

JOHN P. ADAMS, M.D., Professor and Chairman, Department of Orthopedic Surgery, George Washington University Medical Center, Washington, D. C.

JAMES S. BROOME, M.D., Instructor in Orthopedics, Tufts University School of Medicine, Boston, Massachusetts. Chief of Orthopedics, USPHS Hospital, Brighton, Massachusetts.

JOHN F. CONNOLLY, M.D., Professor and Chairman, University of Nebraska College of Medicine, Omaha, Nebraska.

HENRY R. COWELL, M.D., Associate Surgeon-in-Chief and Director of Clinical Research, Alfred I. duPont Institute. Associate Chief of Staff for Research, Veterans Administration Center, Wilmington, Delaware.

BURR H. CURTIS, M.D., Clinical Professor of Orthopedics, Department of Surgery, University of Connecticut Medical Center, Farmington. Medical and Executive Director, Newington Children's Hospital, Newington, Connecticut.

PETER DORNENBURG, M.D., Staff, Department of Orthopedic Surgery, Vanderbilt University, Nashville, Tennessee.

HAROLD K. DUNN, M.D., Associate Professor, Division of Orthopedic Surgery, University of Utah College of Medicine, Salt Lake City. Attending Surgeon, University Hospital, Shriner's Hospital, and Holy Cross Hospital, Salt Lake City, Utah.

DAVID N. DUPUY, M.D., Senior Orthopedic Resident, Charlotte Memorial Hospital and Medical Center, Charlotte, North Carolina.

ROGER J. FERGUSON, M.D., Ph.D., Research Fellow, Orthopedic
Surgery, University of Pittsburgh School of Medicine, Pittsburgh,
Pennsylvania.

JOHN FULLER, M.B.Ch.B., F.R.C.S.(C.), Active Staff, Surrey Memorial Hospital, Surrey, British Columbia, Canada.

NICHOLAS J. GIANNESTRAS, M.D., Associate Clinical Professor,
Department of Surgery, Division of Orthopedics, University of Cin-
cinnati School of Medicine. Director of Foot Clinic, University of
Cincinnati Medical Center. Director of Orthopedic Education, De-
partment of Orthopedics, Good Samaritan Hospital, Cincinnati,
Ohio.

NATHANIEL GOULD, M.D., Chief of Orthopedic Service, Brockton
Hospital, Brockton, Massachusetts. Senior Orthopedic Surgeon,
Massachusetts Hospital School, Canton, Massachusetts.

JAMES H. HARDY, M.D., Clinical Assistant Professor of Orthopedic
Surgery, University of Connecticut Medical Center, Farmington,
Connecticut.

CHARLES F. HEINIG, M.D., Chairman, Department of Orthopedic
Surgery, Charlotte Memorial Hospital and Medical Center, Charlotte, North Carolina.

ROBERT N. HENSINGER, M.D., Associate Professor of Pediatric Orthopedics, University of Michigan, Ann Arbor, Michigan.

RICHARD T. HERRICK, M.D., Fellow in Orthopedic Surgery, Alton
Ochsner Medical Foundation and Ochsner Clinic, New Orleans,
Louisiana.

RONALD C. HILLEGASS, M.D., Assistant Surgeon, Department of
Orthopedics, Rhode Island Hospital, Providence, Rhode Island.

CLAUDE D. HOLMES, JR., M.D., Clinical Professor, Department of
Orthopedic Surgery, and Rehabilitation, University of Miami
School of Medicine. Chairman of Orthopedic Surgery and Rehabili-
tation, Variety Children's Hospital, Miami, Florida.

ARTHUR HOLSTEIN, M.D., Attending Orthopedic Surgeon, Alta
Bates and Herrick Memorial Hospitals, Berkeley, California.

JOHN R. HUCKELL, M.D.C.M., F.R.C.S.(C.), Assistant Clinical Professor, University of Alberta, Edmonton, Alberta, Canada.

ALLEN W. JACKSON, M.D., Attending Orthopedic Surgeon, Northwest Hospital, Seattle, Washington.

RICHARD L. JACOBS, M.D., Professor and Head, Division of Orthopedic Surgery, Albany Medical College, Albany, New York. Attending Orthopedist, Albany Medical Center, Albany, New York.

MELVIN H. JAHSS, M.D., Associate Clinical Professor of Orthopedic Surgery, Mt. Sinai School of Medicine, New York. Attending and Chief of Orthopedic Foot Service, Hospital for Joint Diseases, New York, New York.

VERNER S. JOHNSON, M.D., Associate Professor of Orthopedic Surgery, University of Massachusetts School of Medicine, Worcester. Chief of Orthopedic Surgery, Memorial Hospital, Worcester, Massachusetts.

RICHARD M. KILFOYLE, M.D., Clinical Professor of Orthopedic Surgery and Fractures, Boston University School of Medicine, Boston, Massachusetts; Orthopedic Surgeon in Chief, Carney Hospital and Massachusetts Hospital School, Canton, Massachusetts.

BARNARD KLEIGER, M.D., Attending Orthopedic Surgeon, Hospital for Joint Diseases, New York. Clinical Professor, Mt. Sinai School of Medicine, New York. Visiting Professor, Albert Einstein College of Medicine, Bronx, New York.

GWILYM B. LEWIS, M.D., Attending Orthopedic Surgeon, Alta Bates and Herrick Memorial Hospitals, Berkeley, California. Teaching Staff, Orthopedic Service, Highland General Hospital, Oakland, California.

RALPH T. LIDGE, M.D., Clinical Assistant Professor of Orthopedic Surgery, The Abraham Lincoln School of Medicine, University of Illinois Medical Center, Chicago. Attending Staff, Lutheran General Hospital, Park Ridge, Illinois and Northwest Community Hospital, Arlington Heights, Illinois.

WILLIAM A. LIEBLER, M.D., Attending, Lenox Hill Hospital, New York, New York; Consultant to American Ballet Theater, New York City Ballet, Robert Joffrey, Agnes DeMille, Martha Graham, Alvin Ailey City Dance Co. Team Physician, New York Rangers.

VIRGIL R. MAY, JR., M.D., Clinical Professor of Orthopedic Surgery, Medical College of Virginia, Virginia Commonwealth University, Richmond, Virginia.

JAMES H. McMASTER, M.D., Associate Professor, Orthopedic Surgery, University of Pittsburgh School of Medicine, Pittsburgh, Pennsylvania.

HARRY D. MORRIS, M.D., Clinical Professor of Surgery (Orthopedics), Tulane University School of Medicine, New Orleans, Louisiana. Senior Consultant, Department of Orthopedic Surgery, Alton Ochsner Medical Foundation and Clinic, New Orleans, Louisiana.

ROBERT J. NEVIASER, M.D., Associate Professor of Orthopedic Surgery, George Washington University Medical Center, Washington, D.C.

HERMAN ROBBINS, M.D., Associate Clinical Professor, Mt. Sinai School of Medicine, New York. Director of Orthopedic Surgery, Hospital for Joint Diseases, New York. Chief of Orthopedic Surgery, St. Clare's Hospital, New York, New York.

ROBERT L. SAMILSON, M.D., Clinical Professor of Orthopedic Surgery, University of California School of Medicine, San Francisco. Attending Orthopedist, Children's Hospital, San Francisco, California.

KENT M. SAMUELSON, M.D., Resident in Orthopedic Surgery, University of Utah College of Medicine, LDS and Affiliated Hospitals Orthopedic Residency Program, Salt Lake City, Utah.

KENNETH C. SCHOLZ, M.D., Associate Clinical Professor of Orthopedic Surgery, Texas Tech University School of Medicine, Lubbock, Texas; Staff, Highland Hospital and Methodist Hospital, Lubbock, Texas.

PIERCE E. SCRANTON, JR., M.D., Research Fellow, Orthopedic Surgery, University of Pittsburgh School of Medicine, Pittsburgh, Pennsylvania.

CARL L. WEINERT, JR. M.D., Research Fellow, Orthopedic Surgery, University of Pittsburgh School of Medicine, Pittsburgh, Pennsylvania.

# Preface

In previous decades, knowledge of foot deformities was derived largely from clinical experience with children. Increased longevity, accompanied by the advent of pension protection and improved health care provisions, has been responsible for the creation of a group of older persons with varieties of foot problems and complications vastly different from those encountered in the younger patient. To provide adequate treatment and care for the older patient with foot disorders necessitates expansion of our present knowledge by increased research and clinical study.

The American Orthopaedic Foot Society has been in the forefront in the endeavor to renew interest in the science of the foot. The material presented in *Foot Science*, comprising contributions by members of the Society, reveals this broader dimension of interest which has recently developed.

This volume includes the first authoritative presentation on total ankle replacement. A monumental work on congenital flatfoot is provided as well as chapters on degenerative lesions, industrial injuries, and new diverse surgical procedures for static deformities. Experts and authorities with varied specialities have collaborated in this volume to express the most current and up-to-date opinions and experiences on foot and ankle disorders available in literature today.

JAMES E. BATEMAN, M.D., F.R.C.S.(C.)

*Editor*

# Contents

# Introduction

# The Foot—Present and Future

MELVIN H. JAHSS, M.D.*

The American Orthopaedic Foot Society was organized in 1969 by a small group of orthopedic surgeons foreseeing the need for stimulating and promulgating knowledge in the end organ of weight bearing—the foot. Various committees were formed to organize and develop knowledge in this field at both the graduate and undergraduate levels. We are trying, but with limited success, to initiate foot services throughout the country which, we anticipate, will attract researchers into this field. Our ultimate goal is to educate the public and to provide them with the best foot care at the highest academic and professional level.

In 1973 we became affiliated with the American Academy of Orthopaedic Surgeons, not as a subspecialty, but as a specialty encompassing the growing foot as well as the tremendous and varied problems involving static and degenerative diseases of the adult foot.

What is the present status of both the clinical care of the foot as well as research involving basic unsolved foot problems? Palliative general foot care is more often than not provided by the nonphysician whether it be in the office or at major medical centers. The general practitioner as well as the orthopedic surgeon has little interest or knowledge and in general has shunned responsibility in this field. There are at most three or four orthopedic programs throughout the country that make a serious attempt to teach foot pathology at either the undergraduate or graduate level. There is not one full-time orthopedic residency training program on the foot. There is only one orthopedic foot fellowship available and this position has remained vacant. The American Boards ask but one or two token questions a year about the adult foot and yet the average orthopedist devotes approximately 20 per cent of his practice to foot problems and foot surgery. The foot is not even mentioned by the American Boards as a specific area of interest and competency.

* Associate Clinical Professor of Orthopedic Surgery, Mt. Sinai School of Medicine; New York, New York; Attending and Chief of Orthopedic Foot Service, Hospital for Joint Diseases, New York, New York; Chief of Orthopedic Foot Service, Mt. Sinai Hospital, New York, New York.

What can we anticipate in regard to the future of our specialty? What are some of the serious gaps of knowledge? Let us dissect some of these problems, literally, layer by layer.

The skin of the foot, especially the plantar aspect, consists of a thick layer of dermis, an unusually thick layer of epidermis, and an even thicker layer of orthopedic ignorance. Whereas the protective depth of the skin of the sole is partially determined by the stress of weight bearing, the sole is inherently thick at birth apparently by genetic determination. This thickness is in greater part a result of the overdevelopment of the keratin layer known as the stratum corneum. It is in this specific area that many research dermatologists devote their lives to studying the ultramicroscopic composition, histochemistry, physiology, and chemical processes involving the stratum corneum as well as the process of keratin formation in both normal and pathological conditions. To the orthopedist excessive production of keratin merely signifies the formation of corns and calluses. Yet how many of us comprehend the intricate chemical, anatomical, and physiological mechanisms occurring in the production of callus? Even industry has contributed considerably to the basic research of keratin as found in horns, feathers, and especially wool and fur.

Orthopedists are just beginning to study the grosser biomechanical mechanisms involving weight bearing, including direct pressure, shear, and torque on the sole of the foot. What, however, are the effects of weight bearing on a physiological and subclinical level? It has been shown that simple pinching of the skin causes histochemical changes detected by fluorescein staining. What happens to the smaller vessels of the sole and what is the effect on blood flow with weight bearing? What are the local neurological mechanisms responsible for balance and stance? Pacinian and Ruffini corpuscles and free nerve endings are present in the plantar fascia, tendons, tendon expansions, and joints of the foot and yet their central pathways remain obscure. Since nerve blocking of a toe causes loss of the position sense, we can no longer accept the hypothesis that the stretch reflexes are simply related to their synapses at the musculotendinous junctions in the lower leg, but probably also exist locally as well and are associated there with more delicate and sensitive stretch and pressure mechanisms. It becomes apparent that biomechamics of the foot should not exist as an isolated field but must be integrated with vascular physiology, neuroanatomy, and related basic sciences.

We now dissect one layer deeper, to the fat pads of the foot. The entire English orthopedic literature on the fat pads consists of one small clinical study and a single paragraph is all one usually finds devoted to this area in the larger anatomical texts. What is the exact anatomy, histochemistry, hydraulics, and neurophysiology of these fat pads and their septa? What is their biomechanical function on a cellular or even subcellular level? Why do they atrophy in collagen disease, senescence, and peripheral neuropathies?

We plunge still deeper into the imponderables of the foot—the small muscles and their exact function. What is their relationship to pes cavus? Why do they atrophy with degenerative spinocerebellar and collagen diseases?

We dissect deeper to the bones and joints of the foot. While the accomplished orthopedist may know every tubercle and articular facet of the foot, he is in complete ignorance as to the cause of Sudeck's atrophy as well as Charcot joints and stress fractures as seen in association with diabetic neuropathy and hereditary sensory neuropathies. In patients with neuropathy why do marked bony trophic changes occur completely out of proportion to the often minimal sensory deficit or even in instances when clinical examination is completely normal, including the cerebral appreciation of pain?

It is here that we turn to the research neurologist who, through histochemical techniques on nerve and muscle, is making great strides in diagnosing neuromuscular disorders on a subclinical level. For example, it is now apparent, to the neurologist at least, that most cases of so-called idiopathic pes cavus can be broken down into specific syndromes determined by neurological examination combined with electromyographic, histochemical, and genetic studies. Some patients with neurological foot syndromes may actually be helped by the systemic use of cortisone. It is becoming clearer that not only is muscle function dependent upon humeral nerve transmission but that bone and subcutaneous function is dependent, at least in part, on such neural mechanisms. The marked soft tissue and bone changes seen in causalgia of the foot are typical of the gross effects that neurogenic influence has on these tissues. The effective systemic use of cortisone and sympathetic nerve blocks for minor causalgia and Sudeck's atrophy of the foot reflects the therapeutic application of these neurological relationships to the bone and soft tissue of the foot.

While there are in-depth genetic studies on generalized heritable disorders which may involve the foot, no similar efforts have been made to solve orthopedic problems specifically related to the foot.

Leaving our basic ignorance of the basic sciences related to the foot and its function, we go on to our clinical knowledge. Instead of "yet another hammer toe operation," do we know the exact cause or causes of hammer toes? Why does hammering occur in spinocerebellar diseases, in poliomyelitis with no apparent involvement of the intrinsic muscles, and conversely in poliomyelitis with involvement of the intrinsics? What is the etiology of hypermobile flatfoot or of clubfoot? Can we ever hope to obtain consistently good surgical results, even with tendon transplantation, without being able to determine accurate scientific quantitative measurements of the balance of power between the individual long and short muscles of the foot?

Another critical unexplored clinical area is plastic surgery of the sole of the foot that must be correlated with the unsolved problems of sensory reinnervation, replacement of fat pads, and revascularization.

What then is the future of the Foot Society? In view of the present day orthopedic apathy toward the foot as a specific field of interest, should we rely upon nonorthopedic medical professions, nonmedical foot specialists, or the nonphysician researcher to understand and solve our clinical problems?

I believe the most effective solution will be through the development of a new breed of well trained academic orthopedic surgeon specifically interested in the foot, who will be able to apply basic research to these clinical problems. Such men would most naturally develop as a byproduct of orthopedic foot services at major educational centers. If we are to maintain the care of the foot within the orthopedic domain, it is therefore mandatory that all of us as well as the American Academy of Orthopaedic Surgeons and the American Boards assume responsibility for the rapid development of self-contained orthopedic foot services in its broadest scope at all of our major teaching centers.

I wish to thank my colleagues for the privilege of serving as President of the American Orthopaedic Foot Society, as well as the American Academy of Orthopaedic Surgeons for their continued interest and assistance in our growing foot society.

Melvin H. Jahss, M.D.
President, American Orthopaedic
Foot Society (1973-1974)

*Chapter 1*

# Human Fibular Dynamics*

CARL R. WEINERT, JR., M.D.†

JAMES H. McMASTER, M.D.‡

PIERCE E. SCRANTON, JR., M.D.§

ROGER J. FERGUSON, M.D., PH.D.//

Standard descriptions of ankle anatomy and function are based upon cadaver dissections; literature contains very little information on how the ankle functions dynamically in vivo. We will describe investigations demonstrating motion of the tibiofibular unit during weight bearing which simultaneoulsy maximizes ankle stability and dissipates stress imposed upon the joint.

The tibia and fibula in man are connected by the capsule of the superior tibiofibular joint, the interosseous membrane whose fibers pass inferiorly from the tibia to the fibula, and the ligamentous structures of the inferior tibiofibular syndesmosis.[5, 9] Although these structures provide a firm bond between the tibia and fibula, a small amount of motion must be present to permit normal function of the ankle joint.[1-3, 5] Bromfeild stressed the importance of this motion when he stated that if the lateral malleolus were a part of the tibia and no give or play occurred between the malleoli, no one could take more than a few steps without fracturing a malleolus.[3] This is because the trochlear surface of the talus progressively increases in width anteriorly, so the malleoli, which hug the sides of the talus in plantar flexion, must spread during dorsiflexion to accommodate the wider anterior portion.[5]

---

* Recipient of the Albert E. Klinkicht Award given yearly since 1973 by the American Orthopaedic Foot Society for an outstanding contribution to the furtherance of knowledge and understanding of the foot.

† Research Fellow, Orthopedic Surgery, University of Pittsburgh School of Medicine, Pittsburgh, Pennsylvania.

‡ Associate Professor, Orthopedic Surgery, University of Pittsburgh School Medicine, Pittsburgh, Pennsylvania.

§ Research Fellow, Orthopedic Surgery, University of Pittsburgh School Medicine, Pittsburgh, Pennsylvania.

‖ Research Fellow, Orthopedic Surgery, University of Pittsburgh School of Medicine, Pittsburgh, Pennsylvania.

## ANKLE PHYSIOLOGY

Humphrey, in one of the earliest descriptions of ankle physiology, stated that the change in width of the ankle mortice was dependent on the elasticity of the fibula, which flexed toward the tibia when the lateral malleolus was forced outward.[7] This view was disputed by Nancrede who believed that it was a vertical motion of the fibula that widened the joint.[8] Ashhurst and Bromer agreed with Nancrede, and they also described a small amount of fibular axial rotation.[1] The fibular motions described by these authors were based on examination of non-weight bearing ankles; they did not speculate about the significance of fibular motion during weight bearing.

The accepted descriptions of human ankle mechanics, based on cadaver studies in which movement of bones and ligaments was directly visualized, are summarzied by Cailliet (Fig. 1). "As the ankle dorsiflexes, the wider, anterior portion of the talus wedges the mortice open and the fibula moves superiorly, causing the fibers of the interosseous membrane to become more horizontal. On plantar flexion the narrower posterior portion of the talus allows the fibula to descend and decrease the width of the mortice."[4]

This is an accurate statement of the mechanics of the tibiofibular

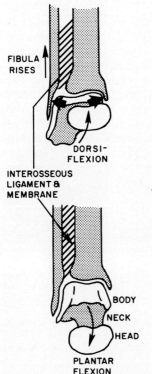

Figure 1.   Theorized fibular movement based on cadaver studies.

unit in the cadaver, as confirmed by numerous dissections. However this would not be a biomechanically sound way for the ankle to function during the stresses of walking and running, when forces across the ankle may rise to several times the body weight. If the fibula moves upward and laterally during weight bearing, the ankle mortice would be most shallow and least stable during the push-off phase of gait, precisely when maximal stability is required. The inconsistency between the descriptions of fibular function based on cadaver studies and the fibular function necessary to provide a stable ankle mortice for weight bearing led us to believe that the fibula played a more important dynamic role than that previously described.

## EXPERIMENTATION

We began by dissecting six cadaver ankles and found that in these specimens the motion of the tibiofibular unit was essentially that described above. It became apparent, though, that only observations on normal living subjects could provide an accurate picture of how the ankle functions during weight bearing. To study tibiofibular dynamics during weight bearing, 16 mm motion pictures were taken of six athletes running barefooted on a football field. Telephoto views of the ankle were taken with the camera lens level with the mortice. Slides made from sequential frames permitted a detailed study of ankle motion at 1/64 second intervals.

In these sequential views deep skin folds appeared beneath the lateral malleolus during weight bearing, suggesting that the fibula was moving downward (Fig. 2). In order to be sure that this was in fact

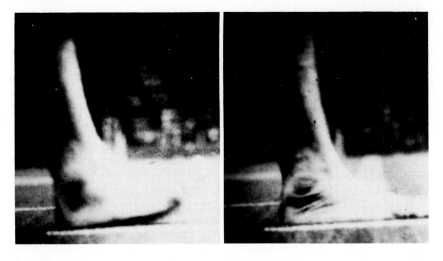

Figure 2. Frames (1/32 second interval) between heel strike and shift of weight to forefoot illustrating the wrinkling of skin beneath the lateral malleolus.

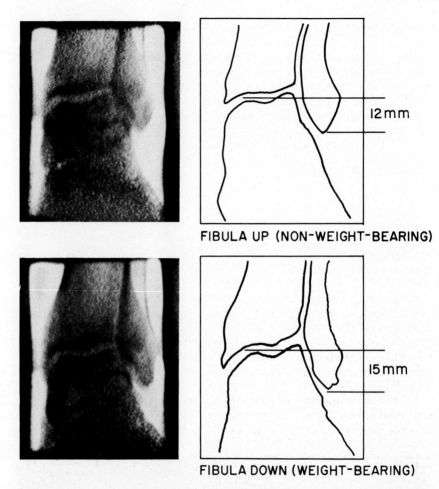

Figure 3. Frames from cineroentgenograms illustrate the extent of fibular motion during weight bearing. (Reproduced from Weinert, C. A., Jr., McMaster, J. H., and Ferguson, R. J.: Dynamic function of the human fibula. Am. J. Anat., *138*: 148, 1973, with permission.)

downward fibular motion rather than compression of the calcaneal fat pad, we repeated these observations using videotape cineroentgenograms of ankles in anteroposterior and lateral planes with the subject running barefooted on a x-ray table. Again the camera axis was carefully centered at the level of the ankle mortice. Two subjects with clinically normal ankles were studied by this technique. Fibular motion was determined from frames of the cineroentgenograms taken with the subject in non-weight bearing and fully weight bearing phases of gait. Measurements were made from the middle of the tibiotalar joint to the tip of the fibula in each position (Fig. 3). The fibula clearly moved distally during weight bearing rather than being passively displaced proximally by force transmitted through the talus.

Because these observations contradicted previous descriptions of fibular function, further studies were deemed necessary. If the fibula did indeed ride up and down on the lateral aspect of the talus, the talar articular cartilage at the talofibular joint should be larger than that of the fibula. Therefore normal ankles from 10 different cadavers were dissected and careful measurements with metric calipers were made of the opposing articulating surfaces of the talus and fibula (Fig. 4). In all of these ankles the talar joint surface was greater than that of the fibula. In fact, in the 10 specimens the longitudinal axis of the talar surface averaged 5.8 mm longer than the opposing fibular surface.

## SUMMARY

In summary, we have demonstrated with telephoto motion pictures and cineroentgenograms of weight bearing and non-weight bearing ankles that the fibula moves downward during the weight bearing phase of gait. This observation was confirmed with further anatomical dissections showing the greater articular surface of the lateral talus compared to that of the opposing fibula.

This downward motion of the fibula during the weight bearing serves to deepen the mortice and provide maximal stability when the ankle is under greatest stress. It also permits some of this force to be dissipated by translating it into tension in the interosseous membrane and tibiofibular ligaments. It is by stretching these structures with downward and lateral motion, rather than by passively moving upward away from the talus, that the fibula can simultaneously provide maximal stability to the ankle mortice and act as a shock absorber to convert compression forces within the joint to tension forces in the ligaments. Far from being a rudimentary strut as some authors suggest, the fibula is clearly vital to normal human ankle function.

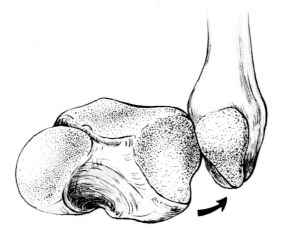

Figure 4. Left anterior oblique view.

# REFERENCES

1. Ashhurst, A.P.C., and Bromer, R.S.: Classification and mechanism of fractures of the leg bones involving the ankles. Arch. Surg., 4:51-129, 1922.

2. Barnett, C.H.: The axis of rotation at the ankle joint in man. Its influence upon the form of the talus and the mobility of the fibula. J. Anat., 86:1-9, 1952.

3. Bromfeild, W.: Chirurgical, Vol. 2. Observations and Cases. London, T. Cadell, 1773, p.78.

4. Caillet, R.: Foot and Ankle Pain. Philadelphia, Davis, 1968.

5. Close, J.R.: Some applications of the functional anatomy of the ankle joint. J. Bone Joint Surg., 38A:761, 1956.

6. Grant, J.C.B.: Method of Anatomy; By Regions, Descriptive and Deductive. Edition 7. Baltimore, Williams & Wilkins Co., 1965.

7. Humphrey, G.M.: Treatise on the Human Skeleton. Cambridge, MacMillian, 1858, p.490.

8. Nancrede, C.B.: An answer to Dr. Randolph Winslow's "Reply" to Dr. Nancrede's paper upon the tibiofibular and ankle joint. Maryland Med. J., 7:76-78, 1880.

9. Romanes, G.J. (Editor): Cunningham's Textbook of Anatomy. London, Oxford University Press, 1964.

*Chapter 2*

# Biomechanics of Flat-Top Talus

KENT M. SAMUELSON, M.D.*

HAROLD K. DUNN, M.D.†

An ankle with a flat-top talus is an abnormal joint in which there has been an alteration of the normal anatomy. In an earlier study of the flat-top talus,[1] a type of ankle motion which appeared markedly abnormal was found in almost one-half of the ankles (Fig. 1). This motion was characterized by gross opening of the joint anteriorly or posteriorly as it went through a range of motion. This was in marked contrast to the gliding motion seen in normal ankle joints and was also quite different from what grossly appeared to be taking place in the other ankles with flat-top tali. In spite of this, these ankles were equally asymptomatic and did not show more evidence of degenerative changes than did similar ankles with a flat-top talus that did not demonstrate this type of motion. This abnormal opening also did not correlate with the degree of flattening.

The lack of significant symptoms or degenerative changes in the ankles with flat-top tali in general, and in those that opened in particular, seemed contrary to what we felt was logical to expect. This was especially so in view of experience with injuries to the ankle in adults which has shown that a significant number develop early and rapidly progressive degenerative changes. In an attempt to better understand this seemingly paradoxical situation the present study was undertaken to examine these ankles from a biomechanical standpoint. It was felt necessary to determine exactly how the tibia was moving relative to the talus and what was taking place within the joint itself at the points of contact. The techniques for performing a biomechanical analysis of the ankle, as well as the results in normal and various abnormal conditions have been well documented by Sammarco, Burstein and Frankel.[2]

They found in their studies on the normal ankle that there is a series of changing instant centers of rotation throughout the range of motion.

* Resident in Orthopedic Surgery. University of Utah College of Medicine, LDS and Affiliated Hospitals Orthopedic Surgery Residency Program, Salt Lake City, Utah.
† Associate Professor, Division of Orthopedic Surgery, University of Utah College of Medicine, Salt Lake City, Utah; Attending Surgeon, University Hospital, Shriners Hospital for Crippled Children, and Holy Cross Hospital, Salt Lake City, Utah.

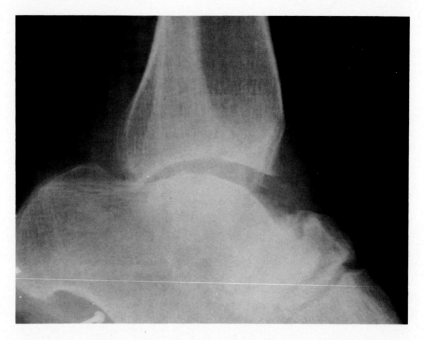

Figure 1.   Roentgenogram of an ankle with a flat-top talus in which there is opening of the joint.

The instant centers were not clustered together and occurred both within and without the body of the talus itself. They also found in non-weight bearing that the surface velocities for almost all ankles indicated gliding to be taking place. Some ankles during weight bearing showed compression and distraction of the joint with extremes of motion, but gliding was the type of motion seen throughout the majority of the range of motion.

## MATERIALS AND METHODS

A number of patients from the original study were contacted and reexamined for the present study. A period of three years elapsed between the two studies. Several types of radiographic examinations were performed during the present investigation. Non-weight bearing lateral views of the ankle were taken at five degree intervals as the joint went through a full, active range of motion. In addition some patients walked with their usual gait in front of a multiple cassette changer with films being taken at a rate of six per second. The films obtained from these two techniques were used to determine the instant centers of rotation and the surface velocities.

Cineroentgenograms were also made of several ankles going through a non-weight bearing, full, active range of motion and weight bearing studies of the joints while the patient walked with his usual gait. The cineroentgenographic studies confirm and quite vividly demonstrate the findings calculated from the other studies. The patients were also questioned again in detail concerning any symptoms or limitations of activities related to their ankles.

## RESULTS

Symptomatically none of the patients had significant symptoms or limitation of activities related to their ankles which was as it had been three years prior to that. There were also no roentgenographic changes in any of the ankles over the three year period. The total range of motion in each of the ankles was also less than in normal ankles.

As had been suggested from the earlier observation of opening of the joint in some ankles, the ankles with flat-top talus can be separated into two groups: those that have apparent separation of the joint surfaces with motion, and those in whom the obviously abnormal motion cannot be detected grossly.

The first group to be considered is that in which no joint separation is apparent. The instant centers of rotation in these ankles were found to lie usually within the talus itself or occasionally below it (Fig. 2). The surface velocities demonstrated basically a gliding motion to be taking place with some mild compression or distraction taking place at the extremes of motion. This was found in both weight bearing and non-weight bearing. These findings are basically quite similar to what has been reported to occur in the normal ankle joint.

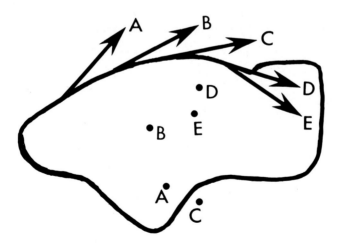

Figure 2.   Instant centers of rotation and surface velocities in a typical ankle with a flat-top talus in which the joint did not open.

While the basic type of motion of the joints within this group was quite similar, significant findings emerged from a critical examination of the gait of patients with this type of joint. The direction of motion varied depending on the gait pattern that had developed for that particular ankle. This variation was well demonstrated in one patient in whom this type ankle was present bilaterally (Fig. 3). In the right ankle the first motion was four degrees of plantar flexion that occurred in the first one-sixth second after heel strike. This was followed by nine degrees of dorsiflexion over the next one-half second during foot flat. There was no ankle motion during heel off and toe off which occupied the next one-third second. In contrast to this, on his opposite side the ankle dorsiflexed three degrees in one-third second as he went from heel strike to foot flat. During the next one-third second the ankle plantar flexed nine degrees as he went from foot flat to toe off.

In spite of the seemingly opposite types of motion in these two ankles they fit a basic pattern and are actually quite similar. The surface velocities demonstrate the motion to be basically of the gliding type with some compression at extremes of motion (Fig. 4). Again this is similar to that seen in normal weight bearing ankles. With their usual gait these ankles went through a range of motion of only nine degrees each. This was in spite of the fact that the ankles had a non-weight bearing range of motion of 27 degrees and 37 degrees respectively. The motion used during the gait was also the most dorsiflexed portion of the non-weight bear-

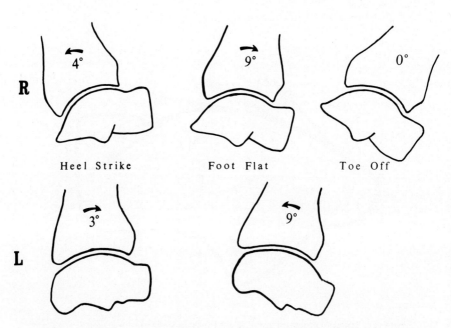

Figure 3.   Diagrammatic representation of gross ankle motion from heel strike to toe off for each ankle in the same patient.

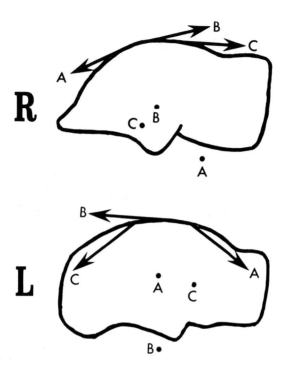

Figure 4. Instant centers of rotation and surface velocities during normal gait for same ankles as shown in Figure 3.

ing gait in that full dorsiflexion with gait produced the same tibiotalar angle as full dorsiflexion in non-weight bearing.

The second group is comprised of those ankles in which separation of the joint surfaces could be demonstrated grossly. In this group a characteristic type of motion also became evident (Fig. 5). In non-weight bearing the instant centers of rotation were usually scattered within the body of the talus although occasionally some were close to the joint line so the distribution of instant centers was quite similar to that seen in normal ankles. The directions of the surface velocities, however, demonstrated a distinguishing and characteristic pattern of motion in these joints. During non-weight bearing the surface velocities showed marked compression and distraction anteriorly and posteriorly. There was usually a small gliding component in mid-range but this was quite small and by far the predominant motion was compression and distraction.

With gait the location of the instant centers changed slightly but this did not appear to be more than occurs in normal ankles. The ankles in

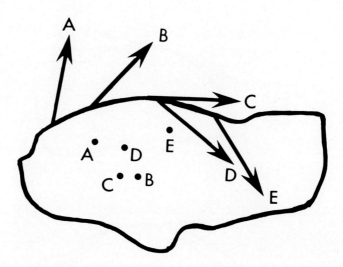

Figure 5. Non-weight bearing instant centers of rotation and surface velocities in a typical ankle which demonstrated opening of the joint.

this group that were examined in their usual gait with the rapid cassette changer and cineroentgenograms demonstrated some unexpected findings. First the full, active non-weight bearing range of motion of these ankles had been determined and this had been confirmed by cineroentgenograms (Fig. 6). Yet with gait the dorsiflexion increased beyond that obtained with active motion and caused the joint to open posteriorly and in one ankle actually produced an air arthrogram in the posterior portion of the joint (Fig. 7). The air arthrogram was present throughout the major portion of his weight bearing gait yet could not be produced while non-weight bearing. His ankle dorsiflexed eight degrees more with gait than was possible to produce in non-weight bearing. His non-weight bearing range of motion was 21 degrees and range of motion with gait was 15 degrees.

Analysis of his gait showed that he lacked normal heel strike and hit the floor first with his toes (Fig. 8). It is probably the lever arm of his foot acting on the ankle that produces the necessary force to cause the joint to open further. In the first one-sixth second of contact of foot with the floor his ankle dorsiflexed 11 degrees and the surface velocity showed compression of the joint anteriorly (Fig. 9). During the next one-sixth second he dorsiflexed four more degrees and continued to compress anteriorly. There was essentially no ankle motion during the next one-third second. During the next one-sixth second he went through toe off and the ankle distracted anteriorly. There was no gliding phase. During gait he used only the anterior portion of the joint and the basic pattern of motion for this end of his range of motion is the same as in non-weight bearing for a similar portion of the range of motion.

Cineroentgenograms of this ankle show it first going through a full, non-weight bearing range of motion. Gross opening of the joint can clearly be seen but there is no evidence of an air arthrogram. The next series shows this same patient walking at his normal gait. The air arthrogram becomes apparent immediately and persists throughout the major portion of weight bearing.

The gait films of this patient show narrowing of the clear space anteriorly with full dorsiflexion (Fig. 10) but this is not apparent on the non-weight bearing films taken for the present study or three years prior and therefore cannot be evaluated regarding change.

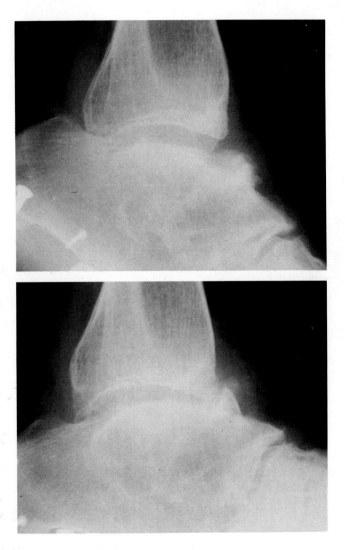

Figure 6.   Roentgenograms showing full non-weight bearing range of motion.

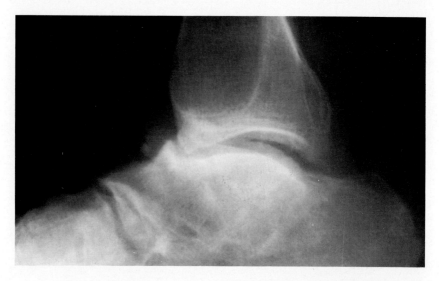

Figure 7.   Same ankle seen in Figure 6 showing air arthrogram appearing during gait.

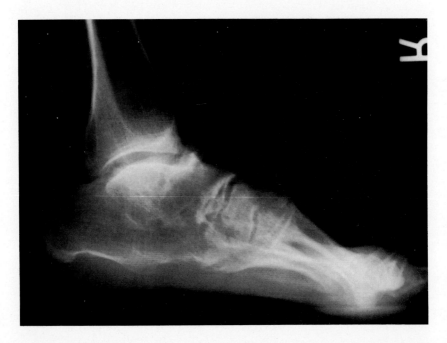

Figure 8.   Same ankle seen in Figure 6 during gait showing toes hitting floor first and absence of heel strike.

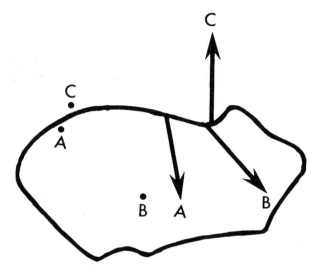

Figure 9.  Instant centers of rotation and surface velocities of same ankle seen in Figure 6 during gait.

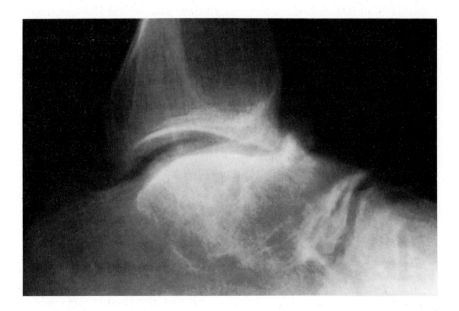

Figure 10.  Narrowing of clear space anteriorly seen only on gait films of same ankle seen in Figure 6.

## DISCUSSION

In investigating the flat-top talus it seems somewhat enigmatic that ankles with such abnormal architecture would not be symptomatic and show more evidence of degenerative changes. This is especially puzzling in view of the rapid changes that often occur in an ankle following injury where the joint has undergone nowhere near the change in contour as these ankles. Several observations about these ankles may be factors in explaining the good clinical appearance of these patients. First, all of those studied with gait films demonstrated an abnormal gait. This abnormal gait pattern was probably established in early childhood and may simply represent a natural protective and compensatory mechanism for the abnormal joints. This is in contrast to the adult who injures his ankle and continues to use basically his normal gait pattern with his now abnormal ankle.

A second consideration is that the range of motion used during gait is decreased from the actual full range of motion of the joint. The significance of this is hard to evaluate. It might be reasonable to assume that this is beneficial in the joints that do not open but would not seem to be as much a factor in the joints that open. In those joints essentially all the motion used during gait is abnormal and the gliding portion present to a small degree in these joints is not used.

A third possible factor is that since the deformity has been present from a very early age the two sides of the joint have had a chance to adapt to each other. It is possible, but certainly not proven, that the internal architecture of the joint may be such that, since it has adapted from early childhood, it might actually be more sound than an ankle with a similar finding that has developed since reaching adulthood.

Probably as a result, at least partially, of the above points all of these ankles have instant centers of rotation that are similar to normal. Also those ankles which do not open have surface velocities that are close to normal. It should not be too surprising then that these ankles function well. Those ankles with joint opening have a pattern of motion that could possibly be called a marked exaggeration of normal. That is, there is usually a small gliding component in mid-cycle. Compression and distraction, while occurring to a greater degree and over a greater area, do occur at the ends of the range of motion. This is in contrast to the abnormal ankles examined by Sammarco et al. They found that when compression and distraction occurred it was unpredictable and often occurred in mid-cycle. Correlating these findings with the clinical picture would suggest that there are certain basic types of motion that are well tolerated by the ankle and others that are not. Marked compression at dorsiflexion and plantar flexion are well tolerated by ankles with flat-top tali. As far as is known there are no other ankle abnormalities that have been described that produce a pattern of motion similar to that seen with flat-top tali. It is difficult then to definitely state whether the ankle in general tolerates this exaggeration of motion or whether only ankles with flat-top talus tolerate it because of the aforementioned or other factors.

## SUMMARY

A biomechanical analysis of the motion in ankles with a flat-top talus was performed. The ankles fit into one of the two basic groups depending on whether or not the joint opened in dorsiflexion or plantar flexion. The first group, ankles that did not open, had instant centers of rotation and surface velocities similar to normal. The second group, in which the joints opened, had instant centers of rotation also similar to those in normal ankles. Surface velocities showed mainly compression or distraction with a small gliding segment at mid-cycle during non-weight bearing. Possible explanations for the good clinical appearance of these patients and the lack of severe degenerative changes in the ankles have been presented.

## REFERENCES

1. Dunn, H. K., and Samuelson, K. M.: Flat-top talus: A long-term report of twenty club feet. J. Bone Joint Surg., 56A:57-62, 1974.

2. Sammarco, G. J., Burstein, A. H., and Frankel, V. H.: Biomechanics of the ankle: A kinematic study. Orthop. Clin. North Amer., 4:75-96, 1973.

*Chapter 3*

# Crescentic Osteotomy
# of the Os Calcis
# for Calcaneocavus Feet

ROBERT L. SAMILSON, M.D.*

A preliminary report on the indications, technique, and five-year results of an operation for calcaneocavus feet is presented in this chapter. The procedure was conceived by the author, and was first performed in 1963. Since that time seven patients (11 feet) have been operated upon, with follow-up ranging from five to 12 years.

## Indications

Crescentic os calcis osteotomy is used in ambulatory patients with symptomatic calcaneocavus feet. It is important to recognize that in a lateral x-ray view of the foot on weight bearing, the calcaneus must be relatively vertical (calcaneal pitch over 30 degrees) and cavus deformity must be present with the apex of the cavus posterior to the midtarsus. The operation does not correct midtarsal or forefoot cavus, but will correct hindfoot cavus (calcaneocavus).

"Calcaneal pitch"[5] is defined as the angle made with the horizontal by a plantar line drawn from the posterior to the anterior calcaneal tuberosity on a weight bearing lateral view. Angles greater than 30 degrees indicate a calcaneus position of the os calcis.

## Procedure

Under tourniquet control, after preparing and draping the patient in the usual manner, an obliquely placed lateral incision over the posterior tuberosity of the os calcis is made posterior to the subtalar joint. The peroneal tendons should be anterior to the posterior portion of the incision. Dissection is carried down to the lateral aspect of the os calcis. The superior portion of the skin incision is about 1½ inches posterior to the inferior end of the incision. The peroneal tendons are identified and are carefully protected. A plantar fasciotomy is performed. A crescentic osteotomy is then made in the calcaneus, posterior to the subtalar joint.

---

* Clinical Professor of Orthopedic Surgery, University of California School of Medicine, San Francisco; Attending Orthopedist, Children's Hospital, San Francisco, California; Former President, American Orthopedic Foot Society.

The osteotomy may be made with a curved blade on a Stryker saw, or by joining multiple drill holes made in the os calcis with a large curved osteotome. The freed posterior tuberosity is shifted posterosuperiorly along the osteotomy line to correct the calcaneocavus. The fragment may be secured with staples or Kirschner wires which are left in place for six weeks. A short leg cast is applied for six weeks, after which unprotected weight bearing is permitted.

## Material

Eleven feet, in seven patients ranging in age from 11 to 31 years, were operated upon. All feet were calcaneocavus preoperatively. Three operations were done in 1963, two in 1964, one in 1966, three in 1968, and two in 1969. For a summary of patient data, please see Table 1.

## Results

All calcaneocavus deformities were corrected. Average calcaneal pitch preoperatively was 41 degrees, and postoperatively was 19.5 degrees. No nonunions occurred. No infections occurred. There was no alteration in triceps surae strength after the procedure. No complications were noted. All patients remained ambulatory at follow-up, which ranged between five and 12 years.

**Table 1.**  *Data on Seven Patients in whom Eleven
Calcaneocavus Feet were Operated Upon**

| PATIENT | SEX | AGE | PREOPERATIVE DIAGNOSIS | DATE OF SURGERY |
|---------|-----|-----|------------------------|-----------------|
| J. DeL. | M | 13 | Idiopathic calcaneocavus feet | 8/21/63 (left foot) |
| J. DeL. | M | 14 | Idiopathic calcaneocavus feet | 12/12/63 (right foot) |
| L. B. | F | 14 | Idiopathic calcaneocavus feet | 11/19/63 (left foot) |
| L. B. | F | 15 | Idiopathic calcaneocavus feet | 9/16/64 (right foot) |
| K. S. | M | 16 | Spastic diplegia with right calcaneocavus foot | 6/23/64 (right foot) |
| L. B. | M | 11 | Spastic quadriplegic with iatrogenic calcaneocavus left foot after tendo-Achillis lengthening | 3/21/66 (left foot) |
| P. H. | F | 11 | Spastic diplegia with bilateral calcaneocavus feet | 3/28/68 (right foot) |
| P. H. | F | 11 | Spastic diplegia with bilateral calcaneocavus feet | 4/26/68 (left foot) |
| D. O. | M | 30 | Spastic diplegia with bilateral calcaneocavus feet | 10/ 2/68 (left foot) |
| D. O. | M | 31 | Spastic diplegia with bilateral calcaneocavus feet | 5/30/69 (right foot) |
| W. McM. | M | 15 | Left hemiplegia with iatrogenic calcaneocavus after tendo-Achillis lengthening | 5/28/69 (left foot) |

* See Figures 1 to 6 for descriptions of individual cases cited in this table.

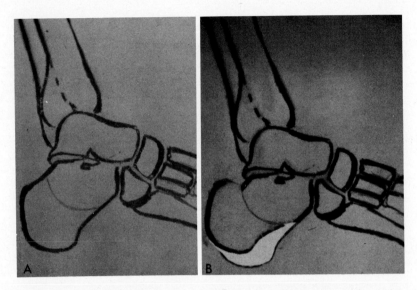

Figure 1. *A*, Crescentic osteotomy of the os calcis. *B*, Crescentic osteotomy of the os calcis; displacement of posterior fragment.

## Discussion

Inman[5] has stated that, "In the so-called normal or average foot, the superincumbent body weight is transmitted through a vertical plane to the talus and thence to the tuberosity of the calcaneus. The axis of the subtalar and ankle joints, when projected onto a transverse plane, intersect in the center of the trochlea. The body of the calcaneus has a medial curve, which brings the tuberosity under the weight bearing line of the

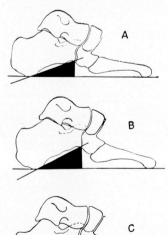

Figure 2. Calcaneal pitch indicates height of foot framework: *A*, low pitch, 10 to 20 degrees; *B*, medium pitch, 20 to 30 degrees; and *C*, high pitch, more than 30 degrees. (Illustration and legend reproduced from Gamble, F. O., and Yale, I.: Clinical Foot Roentgenology. Edition 2. New York, Robert E. Krieger Publishing Co., Inc., 1975, p. 194, with permission.)

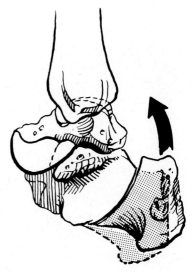

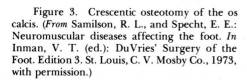

Figure 3. Crescentic osteotomy of the os calcis. (*From* Samilson, R. L., and Specht, E. E.: Neuromuscular diseases affecting the foot. *In* Inman, V. T. (ed.): DuVries' Surgery of the Foot. Edition 3. St. Louis, C. V. Mosby Co., 1973, with permission.)

leg. With such an arrangement a metastable state is created that requires minimal muscular effort to maintain. The variations in the position of the axis of the subtalar joint and the variability of the anatomic structure of the calcaneus may cause the weight bearing line of the leg to fall outside the reaction point on the heel. A momentum is thus created that, if not resisted by muscular effort, will cause the foot either to pronate or supinate. This situation has been recognized for many years and has led to the development and use of shoe modifications and different types of appliances. Surgical procedures designed to bring the weight bearing line of the leg within the reaction point on the heel and thus improve alignment were also devised and are of interest historically. Trendelenburg,[6] in cases of flatfoot, moved the weight bearing line of the leg laterally by carrying out a supramalleolar osteotomy of the tibia and fibula, Gleich[3] osteotomized the calcaneus, moving its superior segment downward and medialward so as to retain the motions of joints and preserve the elasticity of the foot."

Since then, os calcis osteotomy[1] has been used to correct numerous deformities, including varus, pes planus, and cavus. It is only in calcaneocavus deformity that the condition may be corrected firsthand, without masking deformity elsewhere. For example, in varus and valgus problems, the deformity is often in the subtalar joint complex, and the os calcis osteotomy merely creates a compensatory deformity that masks the initial difficulty. One might argue that the deformity of the os calcis in calcaneocavus is secondary to "muscle imbalance," and the crescentic osteotomy serves to mask that "imbalance."

A useful conception of cavus feet has been the following classification: anterior (forefoot) cavus, with the apex of deformity at Chopart's joint may be subdivided into a global form in which the entire transverse arch is involved, or the local form in which only the first metatarsal is plantar flexed; posterior cavus, or calcaneocavus in which there is a ver-

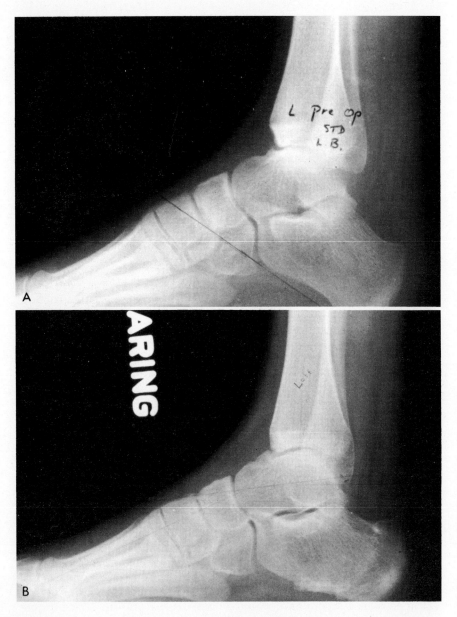

Figure 4.  *A*, L.B.—Calcaneocavus foot preoperatively and *B*, five years postoperatively.

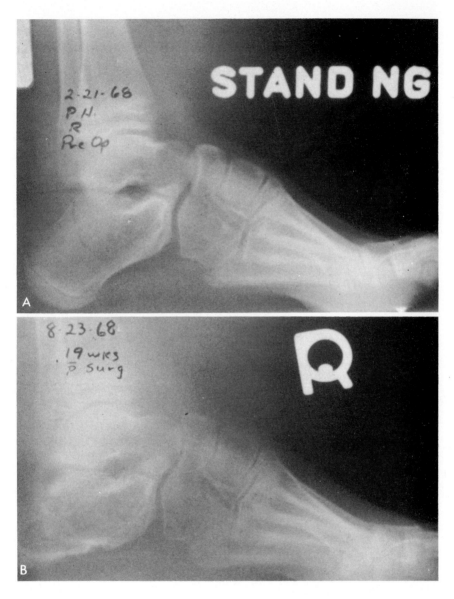

Figure 5. *A*, P.H.—Calcaneocavus foot preoperatively, and *B*, 19 weeks postoperatively.

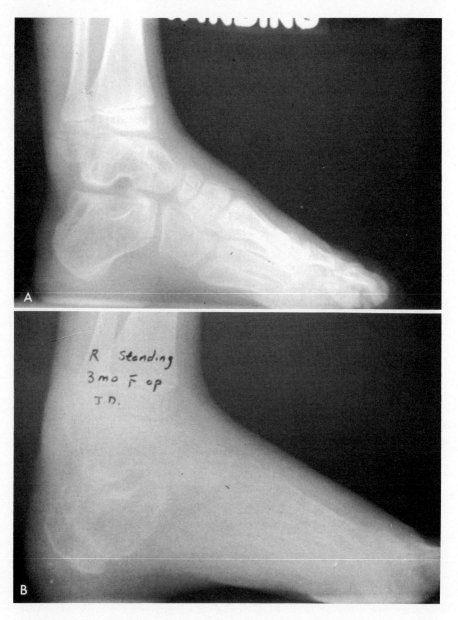

Figure 6. *A*, J. DeL.—Right calcaneocavus foot preoperatively; *B*, three months postoperatively.

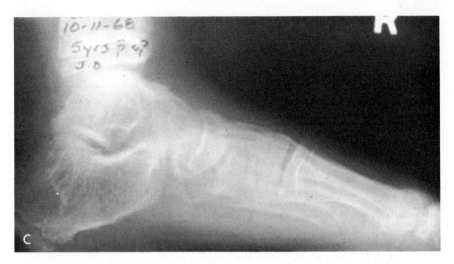

Figure 6 (*Continued*). *C*, J. DeL.—Right calcaneocavus foot five years after crescentic os calcis osteotomy.

tical orientation of the os calcis, rather than primarily forefoot plantar flexion; and combined cavus in which both forefoot plantar flexion and increased vertical calcaneal orientation coexist. It is only in the posterior type of cavus that crescentic osteotomy is indicated alone. We are investigating its use in combined type of cavus, but are not prepared to give our results on combined cavus feet at this time.

## Summary and Conclusions

Eleven feet in seven patients underwent correction of calcaneocavus deformity by crescentic osteotomy of the os calcis. Follow-up ranged from five to 12 years. No complications or nonunions occurred. The procedure is simple, and effective when restricted to calcaneocavus feet.

## REFERENCES

1. Dwyer, F. C.: Osteotomy of the calcaneum for pes cavus. J. Bone Joint Surg., 41*B*:80-86, 1959.
2. Gamble, F. O., and Yale, I.: Clinical Foot Roentgenology. Baltimore, Williams and Wilkins Co. 1966.
3. Gleich, A.: Beitrag zur Operativen Platfussbehandlung. Arch. Klin. Chir., 46:358-362, 1893.
4. Inman, V. T.: DuVries' Surgery of the Foot. Edition 3. St. Louis, C.V. Mosby Co., 1973.
5. Isman, R. E., and Inman, V. T.: Anthropmetric studies of the human foot and
6. Trendelenburg, F.: Ueber Plattfussoperationen. Arch. Klin. Chir., 39:751-755, 1899.

*Chapter 4*

# Naviculectomy For Congenital Vertical Talus

HERMAN ROBBINS, M.D.*

Congenital vertical talus of the foot is a characteristically distinct deformity which has been aptly described as a rocker bottom flatfoot. It is a type of congenital flatfoot associated with vertical placement of the talus and dislocation of the subtalar joint.

Henken, a pupil of Nové-Josserand, published the first complete clinical, roentgenographic, anatomical, and pathological study of this condition in 1914. She called it "pied plat valgus congénital."[6, 9] In 1929 Haglund et al. referred to the condition as "luxation congénital de l'astragale."[9] Rocher and Pouyanne were very descriptive naming it "pied plat congénital par subluxation sous-astragalienne congénitale et orientation verticale de l'astragale."[9, 14] Lamy and Weissman suggested the term "congenital convex pes valgus" in 1939. Their article, which contained an extensive review of worldwide literature on the subject, was the first to be reported in the English literature.[9] In 1956 Osmond-Clarke designated the term currently used to describe this type of foot—congenital vertical talus.[11]

## ANATOMY

The talocalcaneonavicular joint is a synovial joint described as a ball and socket joint. It is truly more of a condyloid joint, elipsoidal in character with a major and minor axis. The ball comprises the head of the talus, which has one anterior facet for the navicular and three inferior facets, two for the anterior and middle articular surfaces of the os calcis, and one for the spring ligament.

The socket consists of three structures: the navicular, the anterior and middle articular surfaces of the os calcis, and the spring ligament (plantar calcaneonavicular ligament). The bones of the socket are strongly bound together by the spring ligament plantarly and the lateral calcaneonavicular portion of the bifurcate ligament laterally, so that while the talus moves with the leg, the rest of the foot moves with the os calcis and the navicular.[19]

* Associate Clinical Professor, Mt. Sinai School of Medicine New York, New York; Director of Orthopedic Surgery, Hospital for Joint Diseases, New York, New York; Chief of Orthopedic Surgery, St. Clare's Hospital, New York, New York.

Congenital vertical talus is essentially a plantar and medial dislocation of the talocalcaneonavicular joint with ensuing secondary contractures of the soft tissues (Fig. 1). This contrasts with clubfoot in which the dislocation of this joint is dorsal and lateral. The deformities associated with vertical talus of the foot are thus opposite those of clubfoot with the exception of equinus of the hindfoot, which is common to both.

## CLINICAL AND RADIOLOGICAL FEATURES

The clinical and radiological features of congenital vertical talus[3-5, 7, 8, 11] consist of rocker bottom foot with prominence of the head of the talus on the medial and plantar aspects of the foot, "Persian slipper foot" (Fig. 2, *A* and *B*). The heel is in equinus. Deep creases are found on the dorsolateral aspect of the foot, anterior and inferior to the lateral malleolus (Fig. 2 *C*). Abduction of the forefoot is produced by a relative lengthening of the medial column of the foot resulting from dislocation of the talocalcaneonavicular joint with secondary adaptive skeletal changes (Fig. 2 *D*).

Other features include plantar displacement and vertical position of the talus producing marked equinus of the talus and, to a lesser extent, equinus of the calcaneus; dislocation of the talocalcaneonavicular joint—the navicular lying on the dorsal aspect of the neck of the talus, wedging it against the os calcis; and forward displacement of the talus relative to the os calcis, with the cuboid remaining in an essentially normal or slightly dorsally displaced position (Fig. 1). The talus has an hour-glass appearance and there is dorsal arching of the tarsometatarsal region (Fig. 1).

In true congenital vertical talus of the foot forced plantar flexion will not reduce the deformity (dislocation) and the first metatarsal will continue to point dorsal to the head of the talus (Fig. 3). Since the

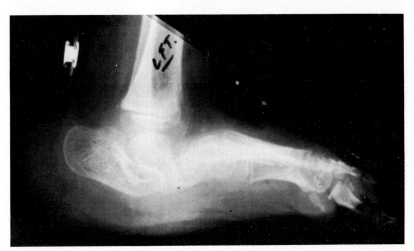

Figure 1. The congenital vertical talus foot is essentially a plantar and medial dislocation of the talocalcaneonavicular joint.

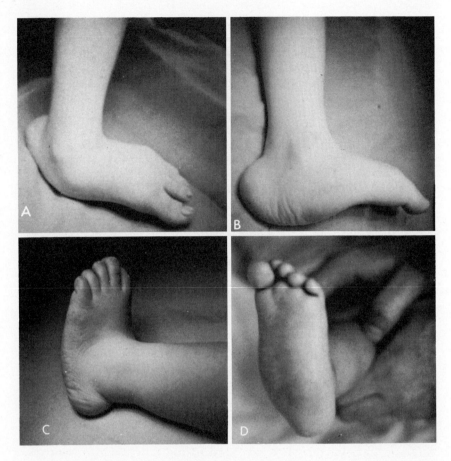

Figure 2. *A*, Rocker bottom with prominence of the head of the talus on the medial and plantar aspects of the foot. *B*, "Persian slipper foot." *C*, Deep crease on the dorsolateral aspect of the foot, anterior and inferior to the lateral malleolus. *D*, Abduction of the forefoot. The medial column of the foot is longer than the lateral column.

navicular is in line with the first metatarsal, it abuts against the dorsum of the neck of the talus, locking the talar head in its dislocated position and preventing its reduction (Fig. 4*A*).

Dorsiflexion does not bring the hindfoot out of equinus, it merely accentuates the rocker bottom (Fig. 4*B*).

Affected children walk with their feet turned outward rolling them into valgus. They have poor balance and an awkward gait.

## ETIOLOGY

In 1932, Bohm proposed that congenital vertical talus is a developmental phenomenon resulting from an arrest in rotational development of the foot at the end of the second or early part of the third fetal month (when the astragalus is vertical). Others view the condition to be hereditary in nature as manifested by the following familial combinations:

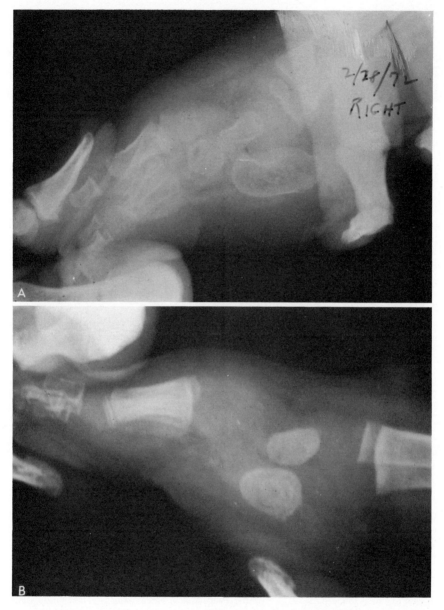

Figure 3. *A*, Eight month old boy with Down's syndrome. Forced plantar flexion will not reduce the dislocation of the talocalcaneonavicular joint of the true congenital vertical talus foot. Note that the first metatarsal points dorsal to the head of the talus. *B*, Two month old girl with unilateral (right) congenital vertical talus. No associated abnormality. The dislocation cannot be reduced.

father and son (Ashner and Engelmann), two brothers (Sigal), identical twins (Armknecht), mother and daughter (Robbins), and mother and son (Lamy).

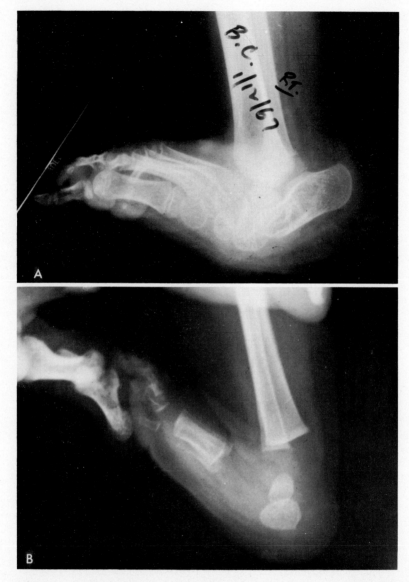

Figure 4. *A*, Navicular abutting against the dorsum of the neck of the talus, wedging it against the os calcis and locking the talar head in its dislocated position. *B*, Dorsiflexion does not bring the hindfoot out of equinus; it merely accentuates the rocker bottom.

Genetic defects in patients with congenital vertical talus have been demonstrated in the form of trisomy 13−15 and, trisomy18;[17] double trisomy (trisomy 18 and triple X);[18] and autosomal trisomy of group 16 −18 chromosomes.

Experimenting on rabbits, Ritsilä came to the conclusion that the primary fault in congenital vertical talus was a deficit in the muscles and other soft tissues. The resultant bony deformities were secondary.[13]

Drennan and Sharrard postulated that an imbalance between a weak tibialis posterior and strong dorsiflexors and evertors is the underlying cause.[2]

It is known that the condition occurs in conjunction with other congenital abnormalities: arthrogryposis (10 of 22 patients),[10] congenital dislocation of the hip, clubfoot, fusion of vertebrae, spina bifida (myelomeningocele, 10 per cent),[15] kyphosis, congenital absence of patella, congenital ankyloses of joints, microcephalia, mongolian idiocy, retardation of intellectual development, hernia, hypospadias, and neurofibromatosis.

While vertically tipped or oblique talus is relatively common, occurring in about 2 to 3 per cent of the population, true congenital vertical talus is most uncommon. It occurs more often in boys than in girls.

## TREATMENT

Treatment should be initiated as soon as possible. If the condition is diagnosed at birth, there may be a chance to achieve and retain reduction of the talocalcaneonavicular joint by closed means. As a rule, however, it is extremely difficult and probably impossible to reduce and maintain the reduction of a true congenital vertical talus in this manner.

Open reduction is the only means of correcting the deformity. Manipulation is useful even if reduction cannot be attained because it stretches the soft tissues, providing a more supple foot when surgery is performed. If the child is over three months of age, the uncorrected deformity should be treated by open reduction.

Many operative procedures have been devised. Lange resected the head and neck of the talus. Rocher released the tight soft tissue elements, reduced the talocalcaneonavicular joint, and maintained the correction with plaster of Paris.[14] Lamy advocated complete astragalectomy.[9] Osmond-Clarke did an open reduction and used the peroneus brevis as a dynamic force to retain the reduction by passing the tendon through a tunnel in the neck of the talus and reattaching it to itself.[11] In the proceedings of the Royal Society of Medicine, Stone, reporting for Lloyd-Roberts, described a naviculectomy performed on a 27 month old child with congenital vertical talus.[16] Eyre-Brook did a partial naviculectomy.[3] Colton resected the navicular following the technique of Lloyd-Roberts.[1]

In congenital vertical talus the medial column of the foot is longer than the lateral column (Fig. 2D). This results from dislocation of the talocalcaneonavicular joint with contractures of the soft tissues and secondary adaptive skeletal changes. It is apparent that reduction of the subtalar joint and proper alignment of the forefoot in relation to the hindfoot may be obtained only by reducing the length of the medial column of the foot. This reduction in length can be accomplished by an excision of the navicular. A release of soft tissue structures would then permit alignment of the foot. This procedure is particularly attractive since there still remains a line of cuneiform bones between the talus and the metatarsals.

**Surgical Procedure**

The procedure is done in one stage through three incisions. By means of a medial incision, the posterior tibial tendon is freed from its insertion into the tuberosity of navicular bone (Fig. 5*A*). Release of tibialis anticus from its insertion is then effected, and, finally, naviculectomy is carried out (Fig.5*B*), carefully preserving the spring ligament.

By use of the dorsolateral (Ollier) incision, release of the contracted soft tissues is effected by lengthening the extensor tendons to the toes (Fig. 5*C*), lengthening the peroneal tendons (longus, brevis, and tertius), and release of the soft tissues in the sinus tarsi and subtalar joint. Care must be taken not to denude the talus of too much of its soft tissue. Otherwise aseptic necrosis of the bone may result.[11] The forefoot and os calcis are then aligned with the talus by plantar flexion and inversion. It is usually necessary to do the posterior release and capsulotomy at this stage to bring up the head of the talus to secure the reduction. The reduction is retained by means of two Kirschner wires, one through the first metatarsal and medial cuneiform into the head and neck of the talus and the second through the os calcis into the neck of the talus (Fig. 5*D*).

In the posterior incision the tendo Achillis is lengthened and posterior capsulotomy of ankle joint and the subtalar (talocalcaneal) joint is carried out (Fig. 5*D*).[19]

The foot is placed in an inverted position. The elongated spring ligament is tightened and sutured to the plantar surface of the medial cuneiform bone. Next, the tendon of the tibialis anticus is passed around the medial aspect of the head and neck of the talus and sutured under tension to the plantar aspect of the spring ligament. The tendon of the tibialis posticus is then attached to the plantar surface of the spring ligament and the medial cuneiform bone. Thus, the tibialis anticus and posticus are used as dynamic supports of the reduced head of the talus. Finally, closure of the three incisions is effected, and a long leg plaster of Paris cast is applied to maintain the corrected position. The cast is applied for 10 weeks, at which time it is removed and the Kirschner wires are withdrawn. The patient is permitted to ambulate as soon thereafter as possible.

## CLINICAL EXPERIENCE

Six patients ranging in age from three months to six and one-half years were treated at the Hospital for Joint Diseases for congenital vertical tali (Table 1). The sexes were equally divided. Three boys and two girls had bilateral vertical tali; in the third girl, only the right foot was affected—a total of 11 feet.

Other abnormalities, such as arthrogryposis, mongoloid idiocy, and mental retardation, were present in three of the six patients (two boys and one girl). The other three exhibited no apparent associated abnormalities. The mother of one of the girls also had bilateral vertical tali with rigid painful feet. Neither mother nor daughter had other abnormalities. The first patient was a girl, six and one-half years of age, with

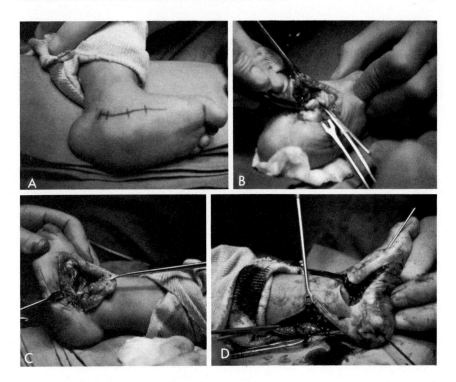

Figure 5. *A*, Medial incision. *B*, Naviculectomy. *C*, Dorsolateral incision. *D*, Retention of the reduction by means of two Kirschner wires.

arthrogryposis. In addition to congenital vertical tali, she had multiple deformities consisting of congenital dislocation of both hips, a short webbed neck, and multiple contractures. The hips were reduced at an earlier age — the left by closed means, the right by open reduction (Fig. 6*A*).

Both feet were rigid and each presented the characteristic "Persian slipper foot." A marked rocker bottom, equinus of the heel, abduction of the forefoot, and prominence of the talus on the medial and plantar aspects of the foot were present bilaterally (Figs. 2 and 6*B*).

The feet were operated upon and postoperative courses were uneventful. After a follow-up period of five and one-half years, the patient has two normal appearing feet (Fig. 7). Motion ranging between 10 degrees of dorsiflexion and 30 degrees of plantar flexion is possible bilaterally, but there is practically no inversion or eversion of the feet. The heel is in neutral position (Fig. 7*D*). The forefeet are straight and, apparently, the loss of the navicular has not caused the forefoot to swing into metatarsus adductus (Fig. 7*A*). The patient has no pain on walking or weight bearing.

The second patient was a 27 month old girl whose mother also had bilateral vertical tali (Table 1; Fig. 8*A*). Although both feet had a normal appearance postoperatively, the talus of the child's left foot developed aseptic necrosis (Fig. 8B). This is the only instance of aseptic necrosis in this series, although Osmond-Clarke has mentioned its occurrence. It is the result of extensive denudation of the talus during reduction of the dislocation.

Three children, two boys and one girl, were seen under six months of age; one of these children is a mongoloid idiot. It was not possible to reduce any of these feet by closed means. Following naviculectomies, all of the feet had good alignment and adequate motion.

The final patient, a retarded boy, was recently operated upon at the age of 17 months.

## SUMMARY

Congenital vertical talus of the foot is a relatively uncommon condition. It is found to be frequently associated with many other congenital anomalies, principally arthrogryposis.

The rocker bottom deformity that produces a "Persian slipper" configuration of the foot is a result of plantar and medial dislocation of the head of the talus with associated contractures of the soft tissues.

Reduction of the foot in congenital vertical talus is not possible without an open procedure. This is because the navicular resting against the dorsal apsect of the neck of the talus has firmly locked the dislocated head of the talus into its vertical position. In addition, the medial column of the foot is lengthened as compared with the lateral column.

**Table 1.** *Clinical Experience with Six Patients Ranging in Age from Three Months to Six and One-half Years Treated for Congenital Vertical Tali**

| PATIENT | SEX | SIDE | AGE AT OPERATION | YEAR OF OPERATION | ASSOCIATED ABNORMALITIES |
|---------|-----|------|------------------|-------------------|--------------------------|
| B.C. | Female | Bilateral | 6½ years | 1968 | Arthrogryposis, bilateral congenital dislocation of hip, multiple contractures |
| J.M. | Female | Bilateral | 2¼ years | 1971 | No associated abnormality, possibly hereditary (mother and daughter) |
| S.G. | Male | Bilateral | 1 year | 1972 | Mongolian idiocy |
| W.E. | Male | Bilateral | 6 months | 1970 | No associated abnormality |
| R.F. | Male | Bilateral | 1½ years | 1973 | Retarded |
| E.N. | Female | Right | 3 months | 1973 | No associated abnormality |

* Total of 11 feet.

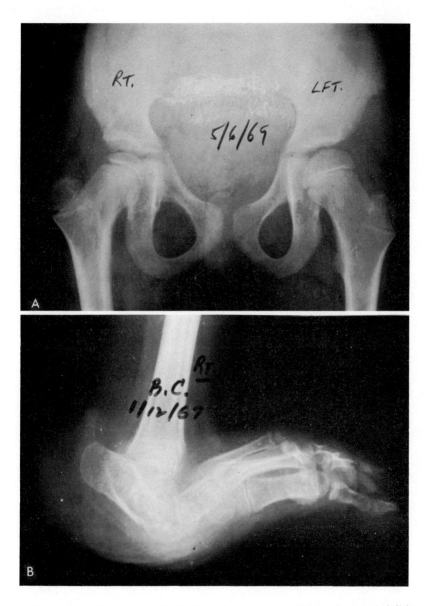

Figure 6.  *A*, Seven year old girl with arthrogryposis and bilateral congenital dislocation of the hip. The left hip was reduced by traction, the right by open reduction. *B*,
Bilateral congenital vertical talus associated with arthrogryposis (same patient seen in *A*).
The patient was six and one-half years old at the time her feet were corrected by naviculectomy.

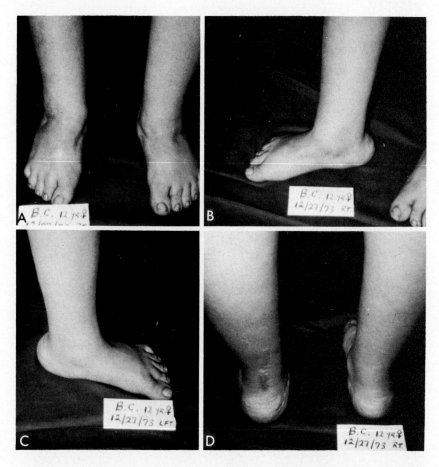

Figure 7. *A* to *C*, The feet (same patient seen in Figure 6) as they appeared five and one-half years postoperatively. *D*, Both heels are in neutral position.

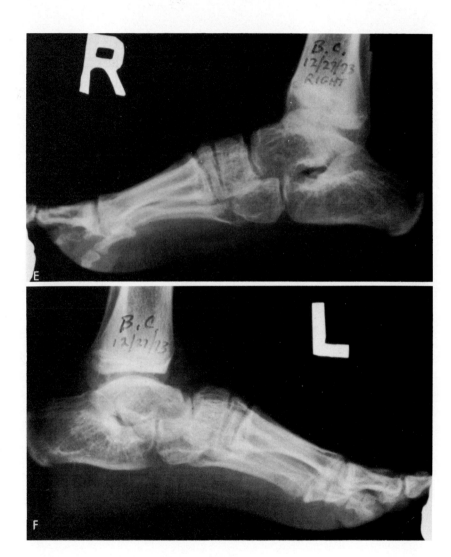

Figure 7 (*Continued*). *E*, Note the absence of navicular. The head of the talus is articulating with the cuneiform bones. *F*, Although operated upon quite late (six and one-half years of age), there were good results bilaterally. The loss of the navicular did not cause forefoot adductus.

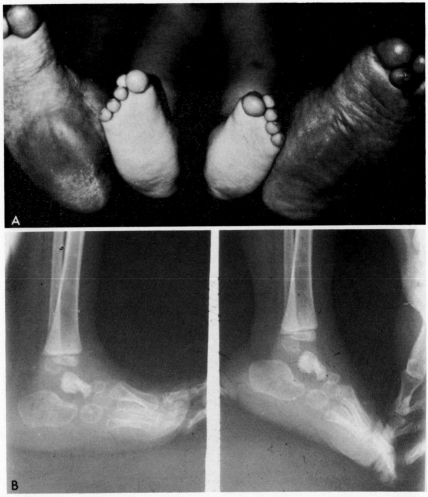

Figure 8. *A*, The feet of a 27 month old girl and her mother. Both had congenital vertical talus, bilaterally. No other associated abnormalities were detected in either mother or daughter. *B*, Aseptic necrosis of the child's talus following naviculectomy. This is the only patient with aseptic necrosis of the 11 feet upon which a naviculectomy had been performed.

Reduction and alignment of the talus can only be secured and maintained by extensive soft tissue release and by reducing the length of the medial column.

Excision of the navicular effectively reduces the length of the medial column and facilitates the reduction. The tibialis anticus and posticus are then used to dynamically support the reduced head of the talus.

In the patients followed, loss of the navicular did not produce an adduction of the forefoot.

## REFERENCES

1. Colton, C.L.: The surgical management of congenital vertical talus. J. Bone Joint Surg., 55B:566-574, 1973.

2. Drennan, J. C., and Sharrard, W. J. W.: The pathological anatomy of convex pes valgus. J. Bone Joint Surg., 53B:455-461, 1971.

3. Eyre-Brook, A. L.: Congenital vertical talus. J. Bone Joint Surg., 49B:618-627, 1967.

4. Giannestras, N. J.: Foot Disorders—Medical and Surgical Management. Philadelphia, Lea and Febiger, 1967, pp. 156-176.

5. Hark, F. W.: Rocker foot due to congenital subluxation of the talus. J. Bone Joint Surg., 32A:344-350, 1950.

6. Henken, R.: Contribution á l'étude des formes osseuses du pied plat valgus congénital, Theses de Lyon, 1914.

7. Herndon, C. H., and Heyman, C. H.: Problems in the recognition and treatment of congenital convex pes valgus. J. Bone Joint Surg., 45A:413-429, 1963.

8. Hughes, J. R.: Congenital vertical talus. J. Bone Joint Surg., 39B:580-581, 1957.

9. Lamy, L., and Weissman, L.: Congenital convex pes valgus. J. Bone Joint Surg., 21:79-91, 1939.

10. Lloyd-Roberts, G. C., and Spence, A. J.: Congenital vertical talus. J. Bone Joint Surg., 40B:33-41, 1958.

11. Osmond-Clarke, H.: Congenital vertical talus. J. Bone Joint Surg., 38B:334-341, 1956.

12. Patterson, W. R., Fritz, D. A., and Smith, W. S.: The pathological anatomy of congenital convex pes valgus. J. Bone Joint Surg., 50A:458-466, 1968.

13. Ritsilä, V. A.: Talipes equinovarus and vertical talus produced experimentally in newborn rabbits. Acta Orthop. Scand., Suppl. 121, Copenhagen, Munksgaard, 1969.

14. Rocher, H. L., and Pouyanne, L.: Pied plat congénital par subluxation sous-astragalienne congénitale et orientation verticale de l'astragale. Bordeau Chir., 5:249, 1934.

15. Sharrard, W. J. W., and Grosfield, I.: The management of deformity and paralysis of the foot in myelomeningocele. J. Bone Joint Surg., 50B:456-465, 1968.

16. Stone, K. H.: Congenital vertical talus: A new operation. Proc. Roy. Soc. Med.,56:12, 1963.

17. Townes, P. L., DeHart, G. K., Hecht, F., et al.: Trisomy 13-15 in a male infant. J. Pediat., 60:528, 1962.

18. Uchida, I. A., Lewis, A. J., Bowman, J. M., et al.: A case of double trisomy: Trisomy no. 18 and triple-x. J. Pediat., 60:498, 1962.

19. Warwick, R., and Williams, P. L. (Editors): Gray's Anatomy. Editon 35. Philadelphia, W. B. Saunders Co., 1973.

*Chapter 5*

# The Relationship of Clubfoot to Congenital Annular Bands

HENRY R. COWELL, M.D.*

ROBERT N. HENSINGER, M.D.†

Congenital annular constricting bands of the extremities are rare congenital deformities that are regularly accompanied by other orthopedic abnormalities including congenital amputation, distal syndactyly, and clubfoot. The associated findings in 25 patients with this condition, treated by the authors at the Alfred I. du Pont Institute, show how these findings are related to the congenital bands and their treatment in children is discussed.

J. B. von Helmont[18] first reported a child who was born with a healed congenital amputation of the arm in 1652. He surmised that this amputation occurred because the mother saw a soldier with an amputated arm during her pregnancy. This early confusion in the etiology of the condition has remained until the present time. The association of clubbing of the feet with congenital amputation was first reported by Bartholini[2] in 1673. Montgomery[10] reported threads attached to the extremities in 1832 which appeared as "complete ligatures about the arms and two-thirds of the leg." These bands made a constriction of the leg but left the skin intact. Martin in 1850[9], and Braun in 1854[3, 4] discussed the possibility of amputations in the fetus being secondary to trauma to the mother in early pregnancy and Braun[5] in his report in 1865 first conceived the idea that these amputations and the strings found entwined about the parts were secondary to a simple rupture of the amnion. Microscopic evidence of the amnionic nature of these bands was presented by Latta[8] in 1925. Despite these and numerous other papers which reported delivery of the amputated parts along with the fetus, other authors have attempted to show that these congenital amputations and bands are secondary to focal dysplasia of the fetus. Streeter's[12] theory of the focal deficiencies in fetal tissue which was published in 1930, continues to be accepted today despite all the evidence to the

* Associate Surgeon-in-Chief and Director of Clinical Research, Alfred I. duPont Institute and Associate Chief of Staff for Research, Veterans Administration Center, Wilmington, Delaware.
† Associate Professor of Pediatric Orthopedics, University of Michigan, Ann Arbor, Michigan.

contrary. Torpin[13-17] has substantiated the role of the amnion in the production of the congenital bands in numerous publications. He has reported on the dissection of 14 placentas (in an excellent monograph) and documented amnionic bands in these patients. Despite the fact that other authors[1, 7] have confirmed these findings, the etiology of congenital annular bands continues to be questioned by many individuals.

## MATERIALS AND METHODS

All patients in this series had congenital bands of one or more extremities. Clinical findings and history substantiate the theory that congenital bands are secondary to premature rupture of the amnionic sac.

Sixteen individuals presented with congenital amputation. Fourteen had amputations of the fingers with six having bilateral loss of one or more digits. Only two individuals had loss of the thumb. Nine individuals had loss of one or more toes and eight of these had loss of the great toe (Fig. 1). Five had bilateral loss of the great toe. One individual had a loss of the entire lower extremity in the midthigh region.

Nine individuals in this series showed distal syndactyly with eight individuals having syndactyly of the fingers but only two individuals having syndactyly of the toes. Several individuals had syndactyly at the same level that they had an amputation of an adjacent digit. The syndactyly was distal in nature with several children having an open space between the fingers proximal to the distal syndactyly (Fig. 2).

In this series, 14 (56 per cent) had clubbing of the feet. Seven individuals had a clubfoot on the left, five individuals had a clubfoot on the right, and two individuals had bilateral clubbing. This clubbing of the foot was not related either to the number of extremities involved with amnionic

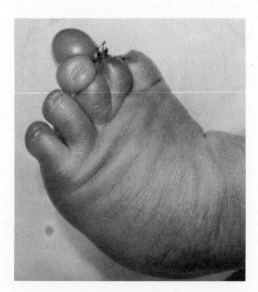

Figure 1. Congenital absence of the great toe.

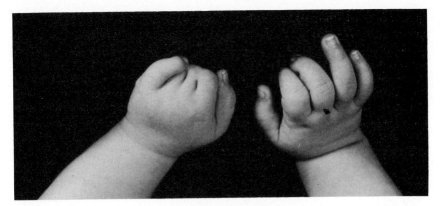

Figure 2.    Open space between the fingers proximal to the distal syndactyly is evident.

bands or to the location of the bands. Six individuals had one extremity involved with a band and three of these had a clubfoot. Seven patients had two extremities involved with bands and four of these had a clubfoot. Seven patients had three extremities involved with bands and five of these had clubfeet (four unilateral, one bilateral). Five patients had all four extremities involved with bands and only two of these had clubfeet (one unilateral, one bilateral). Six had bilateral bands of the lower extremities. Of these, five had a unilateral clubfoot and only one had bilateral clubfeet. Four individuals had unilateral bands of the lower extremities. In two of these, the clubfoot was on the ipsilateral side and in one patient on the contralateral side. One child with unilateral bands had bilateral clubfeet. Four individuals with unilateral clubfeet had no bands in the legs but did have congenital bands on the arms. Of the 14 children with clubfeet, only two had clubbing that could have been neurogenic secondary to the band. The remaining children had clubbing of a positional nature and a typical

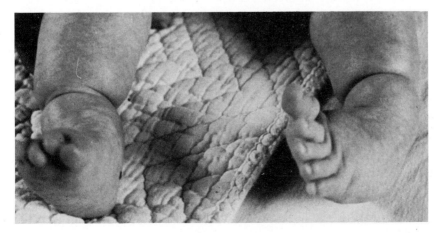

Figure 3.    Typical appearance of clubfeet.

appearance of idiopathic clubfeet (Fig. 3). Their treatment and the response to it was similar to that found in idiopathic clubfeet.

More than half of the mothers had some form of difficulty during pregnancy. Six mothers reported rupture of the membranes with leaking of either fluid or blood early in pregnancy. Seven individuals were born prematurely and two mothers had surgery during the early phase of their pregnancy. One mother had a severe urinary tract infection. There was one history of a strangulated twin. One individual was born post term and one was delivered by cesarean section. Two mothers had a history of multiple previous miscarriages.


## TREATMENT

In this series, five individuals had a release of the band at less than four months of age. Six were released between four and six months, six between seven and 12 months and four had release after 12 months of age. Four individuals did not require release of bands. Early release with a Z plasty repair should be considered in individuals in whom the band is open at birth. Early release with repair of the open defect allows preservation of the part and was carried out in one individual in the series at two days of age.

Excision of the band must be performed down to and including the fascia. No constricting bands of fascia should remain once the band is excised. The entire band must be excised back to normal skin on either side of the band. Following release, a Z plasty is used to allow resuturing of the skin. If release is performed at several days of age because of an open band, the entire open area may be excised and Z plasty carried out. When release is performed on a band where skin is intact, the amount of band removed should involve only one-half to two-thirds of the circumference of the extremity. Release of the remainder of the band, if necessary, may be carried out three to four months following the original release once lymphatic drainage has been reestablished.

Release for swelling distal to the band is indicated only when bony parts are present. When sufficient bone and other soft tissue is present distal to the band, release of the band is indicated even in small digits at an early age rather than allowing the part to go on to amputation. Release of distal syndactyly is indicated in order to improve function of the digits and to prevent deformity with growth.

Treatment of the associated clubfoot should begin immediately after birth. Treatment with taping and casting was carried out in these individuals in a similar manner to the treatment used in idiopathic clubfeet. Two individuals with minor bands of the extremities required heel cord lengthenings. Two other individuals underwent heel cord lengthening at the time that the band was released which was accomplished through the same incision. The majority of the clubfeet were treated with serial casting with repeated cast change until correction was obtained following which a short leg night brace was used to maintain correction.

## DISCUSSION

Despite the fact that numerous authors have reported on the findings of amputated fetal parts with associated amnionic bands and the findings of abnormality of the placenta and have documented these abnormalities both grossly and microscopically, the concept of these deformities being secondary to early rupture of the amnion has not been completely accepted. Torpin[14] has outlined the mechanism of rupture of the amnion with subsequent oligohydramnios in detail. He points out that while the amnion may rupture, the chorion may remain intact with a resultant loss of amnionic fluid without complication to pregnancy. Following this amnionic rupture, which may be secondary to trauma early in pregnancy as has been recorded by numerous authors, the amnion may form strings that are free floating and that may encircle the extremities, the cord, or even the neck.

The findings in this group of children born with congenital amnionic bands show a constellation of abnormalities that is secondary to these bands. All of the findings in these children are well explained mechanically by rupture of the amnionic membrane with loss of the amnionic fluid and the formation of amnionic bands that encircle the extremities. A review of the amputations found in these children shows that 14 had amputations in the hands with six having bilateral loss of one or more digits but with only two individuals having a loss of the thumb. This is readily explained by the fact that the thumb is kept clasped in the palm during gestation and therefore, a mechanical entrapment of the thumb by the bands is less likely than a mechanical entrapment of the digits. In addition, the great toe was lost in eight individuals with five having bilateral loss of the great toes. Again, one would expect the great toe to be involved more often mechanically than the other toes because of the small size of the other toes and the fact that the great toe is held abducted from the foot in the fetus.

The high incidence of distal syndactyly, with several individuals showing a picture of open clefts between the digits proximal to the area where the fingers are tied together distally, supports the mechanical theory. Several individuals had syndactyly of digits at the same level that an adjacent digit was amputated, presumably by the same constricting band.

The high incidence of clubbing of the feet in this series — 56 per cent — can also be explained on the basis of oligohydramnios. DeMyer and Baird[6] have produced clubbing of the paws of rats by removing fluid from the amnionic sac during gestation. Poswillo[11] has shown limb defects in nine of 49 embryos following perforation of the amnion. Six of these rats had ring constriction of the extremities and five had a condition of the limbs similar to clubbing of the feet in man. Three of the rats had syndactyly. Therefore, it is logical to assume that loss of amnionic fluid allows clubbing of the feet secondary to a decrease in the size of the uterine cavity. This substantiates the theory that the entire constellation of abnormalities seen in these children is secondary to early rupture of the amnion.

## SUMMARY

A review of 25 patients with congenital annular bands of the extremities revealed a high incidence of congenital amputations, distal syndactyly, and clubfeet. The clubfeet found in 56 per cent of these individuals should be treated by early manipulation and casting followed by heel cord lengthening if indicated. The etiology of this constellation of abnormalities is early rupture of the amnion with formation of amnionic bands and oligohydramnios. The orthopedic abnormalities found in these individuals are readily explained by this etiologic consideration.

## REFERENCES

1. Baker, C. J., and Rudolph, A. J.: Congenital ring constrictions and intrauterine amputations. Am. J. Dis. Child., *121*:393-400, 1971.
2. Bartholini, T.: De Observationibus Raris Medicorum. Acta Med. et Phil. Hafn., *2*:1-3, 1673.
3. Braun, G.: Uber spontane Amputationen des Foetus und ihre Beziehungen zu den amniotischen Bandern. Z. Ges. Aertz Wien, *2*:185-200, 1854.
4. Braun, G.: Neuer Beitrag zur Lehre von den amniotischen Bandern und deren Einfluss auf die fotale Entwicklung. Med. Jahrb., *4*:3-15, 1862.
5. Braun, G.: Die strangformige Aufwickelung des Amnion um den Nabelstraug des reifen Kindes—eine seltene Ursache des intrauterinen Foetaltodes. Oest. Z. Prakt. Heilk., *11*:181-184, 1865.
6. DeMyer, W., and Baird, I.: Mortality and skeletal malformations from amniocentesis and oligohydramnios in rats: Cleft palate, clubfoot, microstomia, and adactyly. Teratology, *2*:33-37, 1969.
7. Field, J. H., and Krag, D. O.: Congenital constricting bands and congenital amputation of the fingers: Placental studies. J. Bone Joint Surg., *55A*:1035-1041, 1973.
8. Latta, J. S.: Spontaneous intrauterine amputations. Am. J. Obstet. Gynecol., *10*:640-648, 1925.
9. Martin, E.: Ueber die freiwillige Ablosung der Glieder bei Fruchten im Mutterleibe. Jenaische Ann. Phys. Med., *1*:333-358, 1850.
10. Montgomery, F. W.: Observations on the spontaneous amputation of the limbs of the foetus in utero, with an attempt to explain the occasional cause of its production. Am. J. Med. Sci., *21*:218-220, 1832.
11. Poswillo, D.: Observations of fetal posture and causal mechanisms of congenital deformity of palate, mandible, and limbs. J. Dent. Res., *45*:584-596, 1966.
12. Streeter, G. L.: Focal deficiencies in fetal tissues and their relation to intra-uterine amputation. Contrib. Embryol. Carnegie Inst., *22*: 1-44, 1930.
13. Torpin, R.: Amniochorionic mesoblastic fibrous strings and amnionic bands. Am. J. Obstet. Gynecol., *91*:65-75, 1965.
14. Torpin, R.: Fetal Malformations. Springfield, Charles C Thomas, 1968.
15. Torpin, R., and Faulkner, A.: Intrauterine amputation with the missing member found in the fetal membranes. J. Am. Med. Assoc., *198*:185-187, 1966.
16. Torpin, R., Goodman, L., and Gramling, Z. W.: Amnion string swallowed by the fetus. Am. J. Obstet. Gynecol, *90*:829-831, 1964.
17. Torpin, R., and Knoblich, R. R.: Fetal malformations of amniogenic origin. J. Med. Assoc. Georgia, *58*: 126-127, 1969.
18. Van Helmont, J. B.: Of material things injected or cast into the body. *In* Ortus Medicinae Amsterodami, Oriatrike or Physick Refined, 1652, pp. 597-603.

*Chapter 6*

# Congenital Convex Pes Valgus Deformities

JOHN F. CONNOLLY, M.D.*

PETER DORNENBURG, M.D.†

CLAUDE D. HOLMES, JR., M.D.‡

Congenital vertical talus, talonavicular dislocation, or convex pes valgus is a rare cause of foot deformity. Most reports on the subject favor early operative treatment to correct the talonavicular dislocation.[1, 6, 9, 12, 13] However the long term results from both the treated and untreated condition have rarely been reported.[6, 7] During the past 11 years, two adults we have examined and treated for other orthopedic conditions were found incidentally to have asymptomatic congenital vertical tali. These patients prompted us to review the long term results of treatment of congenital vertical talus in the Middle Tennessee Crippled Children's Service. Over the past 17 years, in 16 patients 27 feet have been diagnosed as congenital vertical talus. This study represents a summary of the long term results in these patients to offer further perspective on this fairly infrequent condition.

## DIAGNOSTIC CRITERIA

Our review of the Crippled Children's Service experiences brought to light several patients in whom the diagnosis of rocker bottom deformity or convex pes valgus was open to question. This diagnostic inconsistency may also be discovered in the literature where some patients offered as illustrations of convex pes valgus really do not meet the concise criteria established by Herndon and Heyman[8] and other early investigators[7, 10] of the condition. These criteria include verticality of the talus, verticality of the calcaneus with tightening of the Achilles tendon, pos-

* Professor and Chairman, University of Nebraska College of Medicine, Omaha, Nebraska.
† Staff, Department of Orthopedic Surgery, Vanderbilt University, Nashville, Tennessee.
‡ Clinical Professor, Department of Orthopedic Surgery and Rehabilitation, University of Miami School of Medicine; Chairman of Orthopedic Surgery and Rehabilitation, Variety Children's Hospital, Miami, Florida.

47

terior displacement of the calcaneus resulting in loss of support for the talus, abnormal anterior shape of both the talus and the os calcis, dislocation of the talonavicular joint so that the navicular locks the talus in its vertical position, and, contraction of the anterior tibial, toe extensors, peroneal tendon, and Achilles tendon.

The term "vertical talus" is not equivalent to "convex pes valgus" and places undue emphasis on one radiographic aspect of the condition that may or may not be significant. To determine that a true, rigid convex pes valgus deformity is present, the verticality of the talus and os calcis and the dislocation of the talonavicular joint must persist while the foot is manipulated into plantar flexion and inversion (Fig. 1).[3, 7] Of our present series, in four patients seven feet did not meet these criteria on retrospective review and could not be considered true convex pes valgus deformities.

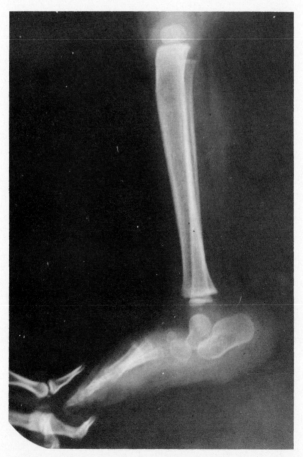

Figure 1. Radiographic diagnosis of congenital convex pes valgus is made if the verticality of the talus and calcaneus and the talonavicular dislocation persist despite manipulation of the forefoot into plantar flexion.

## CLINICAL EXPERIENCE

**Untreated Patients**

Not all of the patients who were disadvantaged enough to lack early orthopedic attention for congenital vertical talus necessarily became disabled adults. This is especially true of the unilateral conditions.

Patient 1 was a 29 year old male laborer, first examined in June, 1962, for a lumbosacral injury sustained while shoveling gravel at a construction job. Physical examination of his back revealed no abnormality although roentgenograms showed a grade I spondylolisthesis of the fifth lumbar on the first sacral vertebra. The patient's right leg was 0.7 cm. shorter than the left, and the right calf circumference was 5 cm. less than the left. The right foot had a medial convexity typical of congenital vertical talus (Fig. 2). Inversion and eversion of the right foot were limited to 40 per cent of the opposite normal foot, and right ankle motion was limited to 20 degrees of plantar flexion and no extension past neutral. The patient stated that his right calf had always been thinner than the left and that he had never injured his right foot which had been flat all of his life. He had experienced occasional aching in his right foot on prolonged standing or walking from about age 17. However he had worked all of his life performing heavy labor without foot trouble. The only real discomfort he experienced from the right foot occurred when he pushed with the sole of the foot against the edge of a shovel.

Roentgenograms demonstrated a congenital talonavicular dislocation of the right foot. This finding, incidental to the patient's chief complaint of backache, did not warrant treatment and over a 10 year period no worsening of symptoms occurred. He continued to perform his work as a furniture mover and later as a plumber's assistant without foot problems. Follow-up roentgenograms of the foot taken 10 years after the initial examination demonstrated an asymptomatic fracture of the navicular where it had been wedged between the talus and the anterior surface of the tibia.

Patient 2 was a 77 year old male, a retired farmer referred to the amputee clinic after a left knee disarticulation was carried out for squamous cell carcinoma secondary to chronic osteomyelitis. He related that he had worked most of his adult life as a farmer and had pronounced flattening of his right foot for as long as he could recollect. The foot had never bothered him until he was forced to bear most of his weight on that side subsequent to his left knee amputation. He then developed a painful callus on the sole of his foot beneath the plantar-flexed calcaneus (Fig. 3). In addition to the equinus of the os calcis, a medially prominent talus and a dorsolateral concavity were consistent with the clinical deformities of congenital vertical talus. The patient had an active range of 10 degrees of plantar flexion and 10 degrees of dorsiflexion in his right ankle but no inversion or eversion of the foot. Sensation in the foot was normal. Roentgenograms demonstrated a subluxation of the talonavicular joint with dorsal displacement of the forefoot and equinus position of the calcaneus characteristic of congenital vertical talus.

The patient was fitted for a prosthesis and the callosity, which was

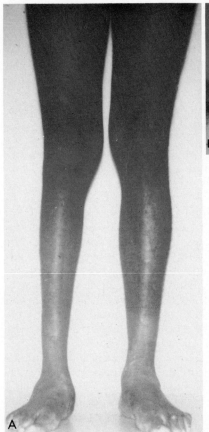
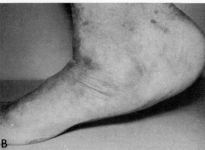

Figure 2. *A*, Patient 1 was a 29 year old laborer with a relatively asymptomatic congenital convex pes valgus deformity diagnosed incidentally during examination for back injury. *B*, Range of plantar flexion.

under the os calcis rather than the medial prominence of the talus, cleared with local treatment. No further difficulties with the foot developed during the subsequent two years of clinical follow-up.

Not all untreated patients remain asymptomatic, especially when the condition is bilateral:

Patient 3 was a 13 year old boy who was examined for the first time because of bilateral congenital vertical tali that became symptomatic and produced aching and stiffness when he first arose in the morning. After he started walking the feet became asymptomatic. However, because of persistent morning stiffness and aching he underwent bilateral triple arthrodeses at the age of 13. The fusions had successfully relieved his foot symptoms when he was last seen at age 15.

**Treated Patients**

OPERATIVE INDICATIONS AND TIMING. The indications and timing for operative correction of congenital flatfeet are somewhat indeterminate both in the literature and in our present series. The objectives of treatment suggested by Herndon and Heyman[8] are primarily to relieve

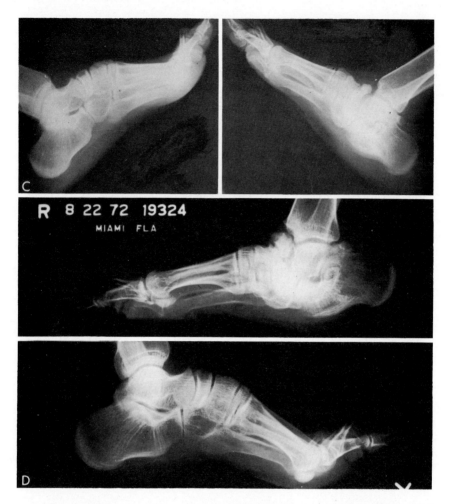

Figure 2 (*Continued*). *C*, Lateral roentgenograms demonstrated congenital pes valgus on the right with normal left foot. *D*, Ten years after initial examination, the patient
still had minimal discomfort in the foot despite the fracture of the navicular wedged
between the tibia and the talus.

awkward gait and to improve shoe wear for the patient. Relief of pain is
not a primary objective since most congenital flatfeet are pain free at
least until adolescence.[5, 8]

Timing of surgery is also variable. Hark[5] described his technique for
open reduction and soft tissue release procedures and felt that complications were more likely to occur if operative correction was performed before the age of five or six. Conversely Hughes[9] later stated that results of
operative treatment in older patients are so unsatisfactory as to warrant
drastic measures at an early age, so that most authors now recommend
reduction of the talonavicular and subtalar joints at the earliest possible
time.

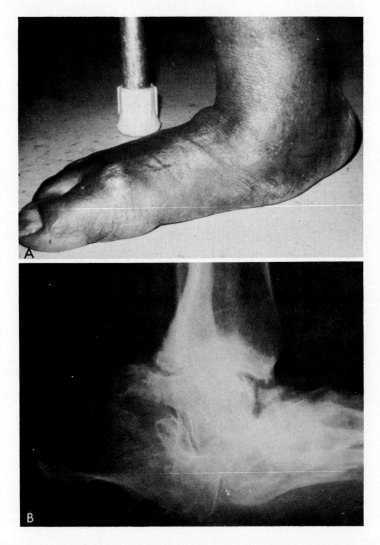

Figure 3. *A*, Patient 2 was a 77 year old farmer seen in the amputee clinic with a history of flatfootedness all of his life. *B*, Lateral roentgenogram was consistent with congenital convex pes valgus.

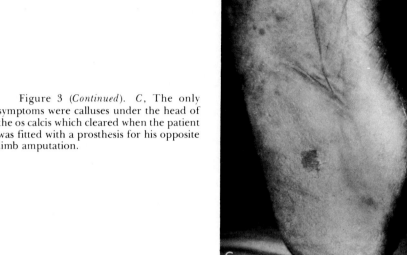

Figure 3 (*Continued*). *C*, The only symptoms were calluses under the head of the os calcis which cleared when the patient was fitted with a prosthesis for his opposite limb amputation.

Indications and timing of treatment are also modified by a high incidence of other deformities associated with congenital flatfoot, ranging in our series from arthrogryposis and congenital dislocation of the hip to sacral agenesis (Table 1).

**Table 1.**  *Abnormalities Associated with Congenital Pes Valgus*

| TYPE OF ABNORMALITY | NUMBER OF PATIENTS |
|---|---|
| Arthrogryposis | 2 |
| Congenital hip dislocations | 2 |
| Absent lumbar vertebra | 1 |
| Sacral agenesis | 1 |
| Congenital shortening of limb | 1 |
| Craniofacial dysostosis | 1 |
| Severe mental retardation | 1 |

In the present review none of the 16 patients had operative correction of the talonavicular dislocation before two years of age, whereas 10 had attempted nonoperative correction of the deformity with casts or splints before one year of age. In four patients six feet showed sufficient improvement with nonoperative treatment that surgical correction was not required. In 12 patients 20 feet were treated by 32 operative procedures to correct deformities. Seventeen feet underwent open reduction and fixation of the talus accomplished by triple joint capsulotomy, extensor tenotomy, and pin fixation of the talonavicular joint. The Achilles tendon was usually lengthened by a separate procedure to correct the verticality of the calcaneus. In addition five triple arthrodeses and one subtalar fusion were performed, either as primary procedures or for recurrent deformities.

END RESULTS OF OPERATIVE TREATMENT.   An evaluation of end results in the 20 feet treated operatively was carried out when the 12 patients ranged in age from nine to 19 years. The most satisfactory results from surgical correction were painless rigid flatfeet produced by either bony or fibrous ankylosis in 14 feet. None of the patients could be considered to have a normal appearing foot or normal mobility of the subtalar joint after open reduction. Maintenance of the corrected talar position after open reduction appeared to be dependent on the development of a rigid subtalar joint.

Patient 4 was a boy treated at the age of two years for unilateral congenital vertical talus by open reduction, pin fixation of the talonavicular joint, and heel cord lengthening. He later underwent a Jones' suspension and interphalangeal fusion of the hallux at eight years of age. When he was seen at 15 years of age he had a satisfactory but stiff flatfoot which was asymptomatic. Roentgenograms showed obliteration of the subtalar joint (Fig. 4).

Open reduction that could not achieve a firm subtalar support for the talus tended to allow recurrence of the talonavicular dislocation. In four patients six feet showed recurrence of vertical talus after open reduction.

Patient 5 was a boy with bilateral convex pes valgus deformities associated with an absent second lumbar vertebra (Fig. 5). Open reduction at two years of age achieved a satisfactory position but at five years a unilateral recurrence was evident. At the age of 10 years the patient's deformity had recurred bilaterally. However, since the patient's heels remained plantigrade and were not vertical, he had no problem with plantar calluses and actually was a better than average basketball player.

Two feet had persistent rocker bottom deformity and plantar calluses resulting from a vertical calcaneus incompletely corrected at the time of triple arthrodeses.

Patient 6 had bilateral congenital convex pes valgus deformity treated by open reduction at two years of age after which the deformities recurred (Fig. 6). Triple arthrodeses were carried out. However the os calcis on the left remained in an equinus position. At the age of 12 the patient still had calluses over the head of the plantar-flexed left calcaneus despite the triple fusion.

A problem in addition to recurrence or persistent deformity after open reduction was clawing of the toes or bunions which developed in five feet and required secondary correction. Incomplete lengthening of the toe extensor tendons after open reduction of the talus produced these toe deformities (Fig. 7).

 END RESULTS OF NONOPERATIVE TREATMENT.   Nonoperative treatment with casts or splints or both was utilized in nonrigid convex pes valgus deformities (Fig. 8) as well as in feet that required soft tissue stretch-

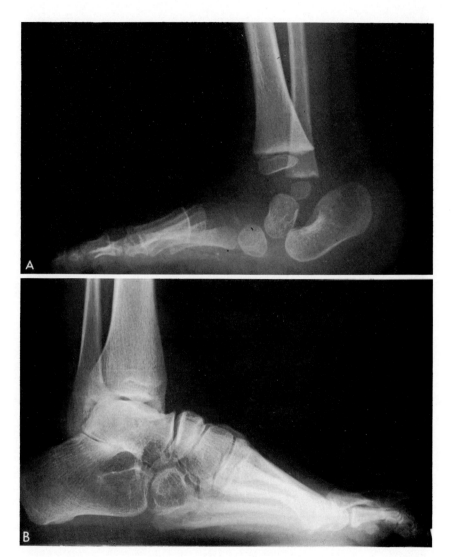

Figure 4. *A*, Patient 4. Lateral roentgenogram showing congenital pes valgus treated by open reduction at two years of age. *B*, Follow-up roentgenogram taken at age 15 showed a rigid subtalar support had developed which allowed the patient good function but a rigid flatfoot.

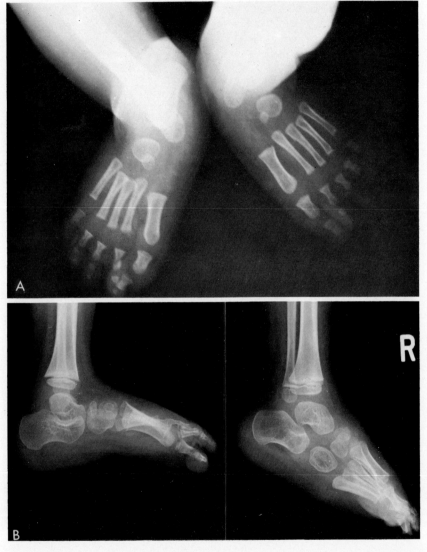

Figure 5. *A*, Patient 5. Anteroposterior roentgenogram taken at two years of age showing bilateral congenital vertical talus. *B*, Open reduction was followed by gradual recurrence of the vertical talus on the right at five years of age.

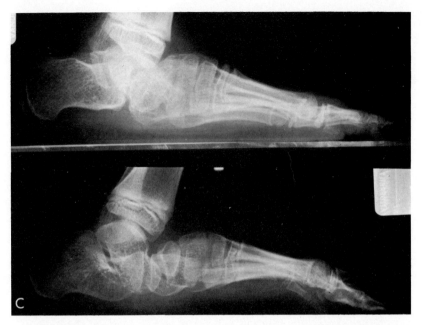

Figure 5 *(Continued)*. *C*, At 10 years of age the patient had recurrent vertical talus on both the right *(upper)* and left foot *(lower)*. His heels remained plantigrade and the patient participated actively in sports.

ing prior to open reduction. Five feet corrected nonoperatively by means of casts and Denis Browne splints showed normal arch and normal subtalar motion on follow up evaluation, and one foot treated nonoperatively became a flexible flatfoot. One foot that was associated with congenital shortening of the limb was treated unsuccessfully by casts and remained in rocker bottom position on follow-up at 11 years of age. Triple arthrodesis is anticipated to offer this patient a better plantigrade foot but presently he does not feel sufficiently in need of operative correction.

## DISCUSSION

The term "vertical talus" has proven to be an unfortunate choice of words that tends to misdirect therapy as well as confuse diagnosis. It is the verticality of the calcaneus that produces the painful convexity on the weight bearing portion of the convex pes valgus. The position of the os calcis must be corrected along with the talus to achieve a satisfactory plantigrade foot.

Soft tissue contractures are of prime importance in producing alterations in the bony architecture of the foot as indicated both experimentally and in anatomic dissection of the feet of newborns. Ritsila[15] showed that a vertical talus could be produced most easily in newborn rabbits by

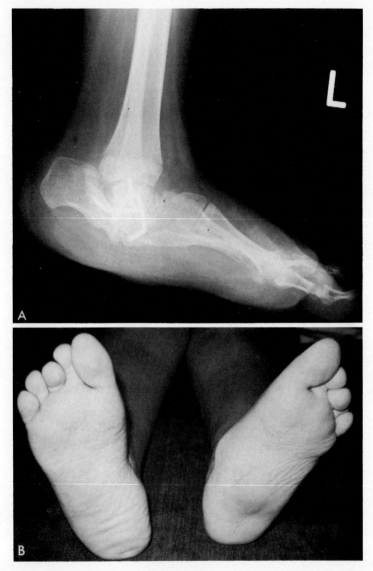

Figure 6.  *A*, Patient 6. Lateral roentgenogram showing equinus position of the cal-caneus which persisted after triple arthrodeses. *B*, At 12 years of age the patient had per-sistent, painful calluses produced by the vertical position of the left calcaneus.

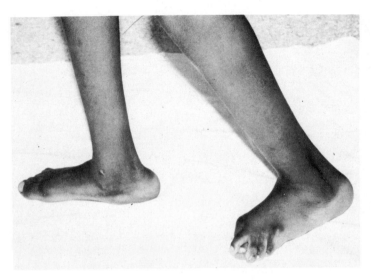

Figure 7.   Incomplete lengthening of toe extensors at the time of open reduction led to bunions or claw toes or both requiring secondary procedures in five feet.


tenodesing the Achilles tendon and surgically contracting the extensor tendons. Patterson and coworkers[14] in anatomic dissection of the deformity have also found that musculotendinous contractures produce the bony abnormality of congenital convex pes valgus.

Any foot in which the diagnosis is questionable or borderline can best be treated by corrective casts or splints with the objective being to correct soft tissue contractures before permanent alteration of bony architecture occurs.[2, 4, 16, 17] Because the initial problem is in the soft tissue rather than bone, treatment with casts or pin fixation to reduce the talonavicular dislocation and reposition the calcaneus works well in the infant's foot.[4, 16, 17] After two years of age the patients who benefited most by open reduction were those with severe bilateral deformities. The following case histories illustrate the types of deformities we think are best treated nonoperatively and operatively:

Patient 7 was a one year old boy who was diagnosed as having congenital vertical talus of the right foot which roentgenographically was quite similar to Case 4 (Figs. 4 and 8). Operative intervention was considered, but on further study we could demonstrate correction of the verticality of both the os calcis and the talus by inverting and plantar flexing the foot, while applying direct pressure to the calcaneus. Consequently the deformity was not considered to be a rigid one. The patient was treated with Denis Browne splints and exercises for eight months as suggested by Regen,[2] while the foot was held in inversion in order to shift the os calcis more directly under the talus. On follow-up

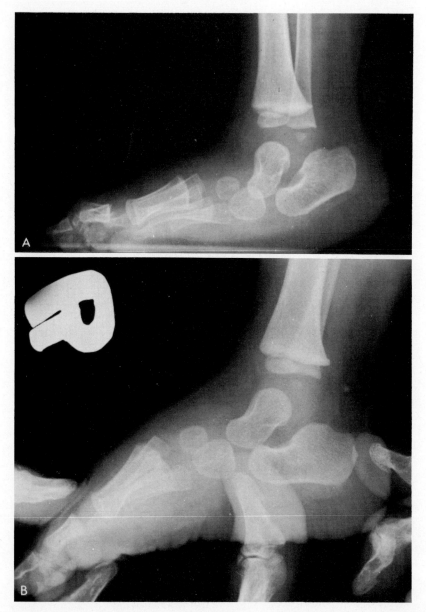

Figure 8. *A*, Patient 7. Lateral roentgenogram taken at one year of age demonstrated unilateral congenital vertical talus similar to that of patient 4 (Fig. 4). *B*,
Lateral roentgenogram demonstrated correction of the talus and the os calcis which was
possible by direct manipulation.

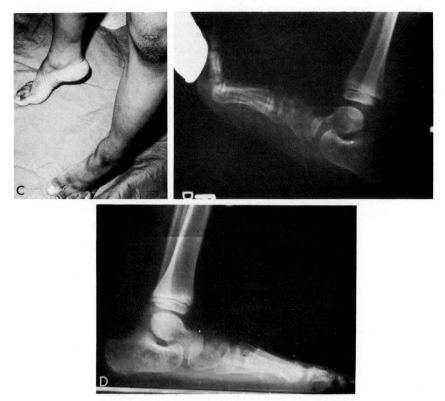

Figure 8 (*Continued*). *C*, At five years of age, after treatment with inverted Denis Browne splints and exercises the patient had a flexible flatfoot. *D*, Lateral roentgenogram taken at five years of age showed slight verticality of the right talus compared with the opposite normal left foot.

at five years of age the boy had essentially a flexible flatfoot. His heel was plantigrade and the talus, although slightly vertical, was not symptomatic.

An additional patient with bilateral convex pes valgus deformities (Fig. 9) and multiple congenital anomalies was treated at one year of age by manipulation and pin fixation of the os calcis under the talus. The pins were removed six weeks later and correction was maintained both clinically and radiographically. Follow-up is inadequate to determine whether the correction will be maintained with active walking but the feet do illustrate the relative ease of correction possible if both the os calcis and talus can be brought into normal relationship early.

At the opposite end of the scale was patient 9 (Fig. 10), a five year old boy, seen in 1966 with multiple congenital anomalies including arthrogryposis and bilateral rigid convex pes valgus deformities. Prior to that time attempts had been unsuccessful to assist this patient in walking with crutches and he remained a nonwalker. Following a series of cast

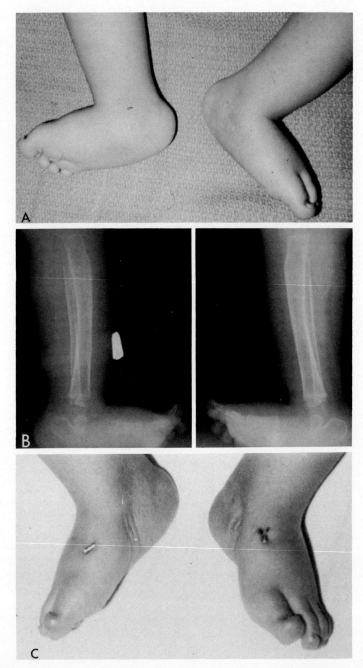

Figure 9. Patient 8. Clinical photograph (*A*) and lateral roentgenogram (*B*) taken at one year of age prior to manipulation and pin fixation of the subtalar and talonavicular joint. *C* and *D*, Clinical photograph and lateral roentgenogram demonstrating correction of vertical talus and os calcis, and pin fixation.

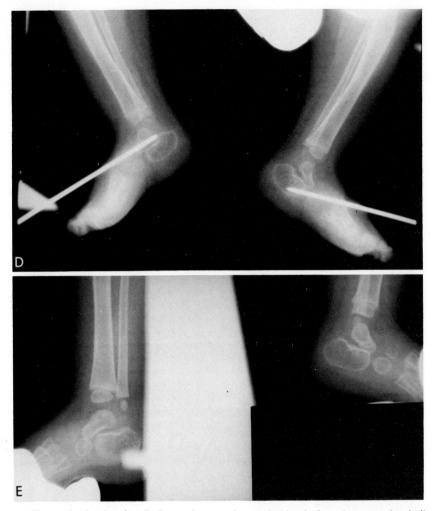

Figure 9 *(Continued)*. *E*, Correction was then maintained after pin removal as indicated by roentgenograms four months following treatment.

applications, bilateral open reductions with soft tissue release of the talonavicular dislocations were performed.

Within five months after correction of the foot deformities, this boy could walk independently on crutches. He has been walking without problems in his feet, which are now rigid flatfeet in plantigrade position, and has maintained this correction for the seven years subsequent to open reduction. Although correction of the severe foot deformities was not the sole factor in allowing this patient to become an independent walker on crutches, the better balance his plantigrade feet allowed him

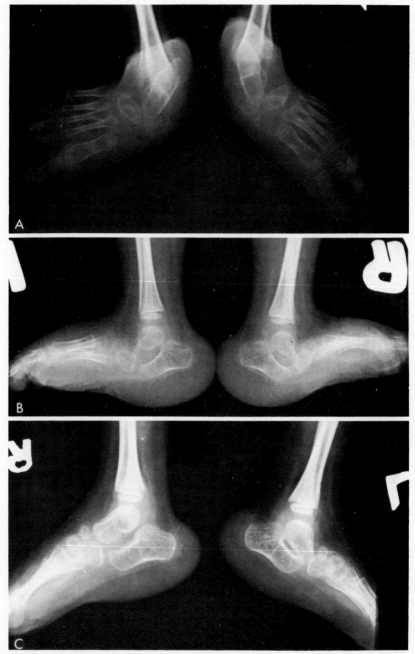

Figure 10.  *A* and *B*, Patient 9. Anteroposterior and lateral roentgenograms showing convex pes valgus deformities in a five year old child with arthrogryposis. *C*, Lateral
roentgenograms after open reduction of feet showed corrected rocker-bottom deformity
which provided the patient with rigid flatfeet that allowed him to become an independent
walker on crutches.

was certainly important. In retrospect earlier operative correction of his feet would have mitigated his struggle to walk.

## SUMMARY

Our review of 18 patients diagnosed as having congenital vertical talus, including two untreated cases in adults, indicates that the radiographic verticality of the talus tends to be overemphasized and the condition overdiagnosed, especially in the young infant's foot. The age of the patient and the varying severity of the condition modify our approach to therapy. A foot with a vertical talus that lacks the other components of a severe convex pes valgus deformity in a young child can be treated nonoperatively to achieve a near normal foot, or a flexible flatfoot. The true convex pes valgus deformity requires early correction. Inversion reduction of the talonavicular and subtalar joints with pin or splint fixation can be effective in children under two years of age.

In our experiences with feet treated by open reduction after two years of age, maintainance of correction depends on development of a rigid subtalar support. The vertical position of the calcaneus is as important to correct as is the vertical talus in order to improve the rocker-bottom deformity of the foot.

## REFERENCES

1. Coleman, S., Stelling, F., and Jarrett, J.: Pathomechanics and treatment of congenital vertical talus. Clin. Orthop., 70:62-72, 1970.

2. Connolly, J., Regen, E., and Hillman, J. W.: Pigeon-toes and flatfeet. Pediat. Clin. North Amer., 17:291-307, 1970.

3. Eyre-Brook, A.: Congenital vertical talus. J. Bone Joint Surg., 49B:618-627, 1967.

4. Giannestras, N.: Recognition and treatment of flatfeet in infancy. Clin. Orthop. 70:10-29, 1970.

5. Hark, F.: Rocker-foot due to congenital subluxation of the talus. J. Bone Joint Surg., 32A:344-350, 1950.

6. Harrold, A. J.: Congenital vertical talus in infancy. J. Bone Joint Surg., 49B:634-643, 1967.

7. Haveson, S.: Congenital flatfoot due to talonavicular dislocations (vertical talus). Radiology, 72:19-25, 1959.

8. Herndon, C., and Heyman, C.: Problems in the recognition and treatment of congenital convex pes valgus. J. Bone Joint Surg., 45A:413-429, 1963.

9. Hughes, J.: Congenital vertical talus. J. Bone Joint Surg., 39B:580, 1957.

10. Lamy, L., and Weissman, L.: Congenital convex pes valgus. J. Bone Joint Surg., 21:79-91, 1939.

11. Lloyd-Roberts, G., and Spence, A.: Congenital vertical talus. J. Bone Joint Surg., 40B:33-41, 1958.

12. Osmond-Clarke, H.: Congenital vertical talus. J. Bone Joint Surg., 38B:334-341, 1956.

13. Osmond-Clarke, H.: Discussion of J. Hughes' paper, Congenital vertical talus. J. Bone Joint Surg., 35B:580, 1957.

14. Patterson, W., Fitz, D., and Smith, W.: The pathologic anatomy of congenital convex pes valgus. J. Bone Joint Surg., *50A*:458-466, 1968.

15. Ritsilä, V.: Talipes equinovarus and vertical talus produced experimentally in newborn rabbits. Acta. Orth. Scand., Suppl. 121, 1968.

16. Silk, F., and Wainwright, D.: The recognition and treatment of congenital flatfoot in infancy. J. Bone Joint Surg., *49B*:628-633, 1967.

17. Storen, H.: Congenital convex pes valgus with vertical talus. Acta. Orth. Scand., Suppl. 94, 1967.

*Chapter 7*

# Flexible Valgus Flatfoot Resulting from Naviculocuneiform and Talonavicular Sag

## *Surgical Correction in the Adolescent*

NICHOLAS J. GIANNESTRAS, M.D.*

"If one has a cut on the finger or a felon, he goes to the hospital and has surgical treatment.

If he has a painful foot, he is subject to ridicule and is sent to the shoe salesman for relief."

**ROYAL WHITMAN**

There are certain types of flatfeet which, in spite of supportive measures for long periods of time, continue to assume severe valgus position with marked flattening of the longitudinal arch upon the cessation of the supportive therapy. These are the feet that are diagnosed as valgus type in young children. These youngsters have continued for eight to 10 years with a history of "weak ankles" or "growing pains," little or no longitudinal arches, and easy fatigability. They are relieved by supportive appliances. However these feet never assume normal position. These flatfeet present a problem of sufficient gravity to challenge our best judgment. One cannot help but agree with Lowman[14] who so succinctly stated, "The fact that many patients with extreme flatfoot go through life without symptoms is not a legitimate excuse for failure to advise corrective surgery. The deformity needs consideration just as much as a clubfoot of similar degree or a foot weakened and deformed

* Associate Clinical Professor, Department of Surgery, Division of Orthopedics, University of Cincinnati School of Medicine; Director of Foot Clinic, University of Cincinnati Medical Center; Director of Orthopedic Education, Department of Orthopedics, Good Samaritan Hospital, Cincinnati, Ohio.

67

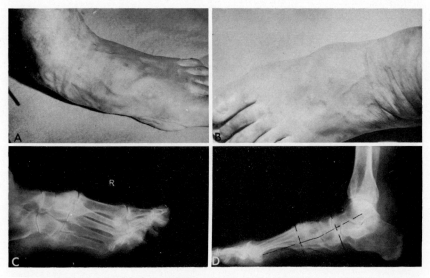

Figure 1. *A*, Adult disabling symptomatic flatfoot unrelieved by various conservative measures. *B*, Exostosis at the metatarsocuneiform joint probably resulting from abnormal stresses placed on this joint because of the flatfoot, resulting in a painful bony prominence in the foot of the same patient seen in *A*. *C*, Roentgenographic evidence of the exostosis and narrowing of the tarsometatarsal joint as a result of degenerative changes in the flatfoot seen in *A*. *D*, Adult symptomatic flatfoot caused by a mild sag of the naviculocuneiform joint. Persistent disability exists in spite of the application of conservative therapeutic measures.

by paralysis." Along the same line of thought one can, by analogy, compare the flatfoot with a structural scoliotic curve of approximately 45 degrees that is surgically corrected to overcome the cosmetic deformity that is present.

Surgical correction of the flexible flatfoot in the adolescent, particularly if only mildly symptomatic, has been a source of controversy. Conservative minded orthopedists believe that flexible flatfeet will, almost invariably, remain symptom-free even under abnormal stresses, and that with corrective shoes or supports any symptomatology can be relieved. This type of thinking has doomed many flatfooted persons to lives of pain and disability (Fig. 1).

The surgical correction of symptomatic flatfoot appears to have been a problem of some magnitude even in the nineteenth century. The patients either learned to live with their anamorphous feet or were treated with strap braces of various types, some of which bore close resemblance to instruments of torture in the late 1800's. With the development of Lister's sterile technique, the orthopedically oriented surgeon began to consider the surgical correction of symptomatic flatfeet as a distinct possibility.

One sees a gradual pattern emerging as the literature is reviewed. Differentiation is made between the valgus flexible flatfoot caused by sag of the naviculocuneiform joint as opposed to plantar **flexion** of the talus. The congenital rigid flatfoot and its therapy are also delineated and differentiated from the type of therapy used for flexible flatfoot deformity. Yet, in spite of almost 100 years of interest in the problems of the flatfoot and its surgical correction when indicated, it has not been until the last 15 years that any meaningful end result studies have been presented and specific surgical techniques for correction have been evolved.

The term flatfoot has been used to describe all foot deformities distinguished by the lowering of the longitudinal arch. Differentiation should be made between the relaxed, clinically flat-appearing foot that shows no roentgenographic evidence of disalignment of the tarsal bones (Fig. 2) and is almost invariably asymptomatic, and the valgus-type flexible flatfoot caused by disalignment of the naviculocuneiform, talonavicular, or talocalcaneal joint or any combination of these three misaligned articulations. It is the author's intent to submit a classification of the various types of flatfeet and one particular operation to correct two of the more common types of flexible valgus flatfoot deformity.

## EMBRYOLOGY OF FOOT DEVELOPMENT

The lower limb buds, although developed slightly later than the upper are, at first, seen in the embryo to be 4 mm in length. At this stage

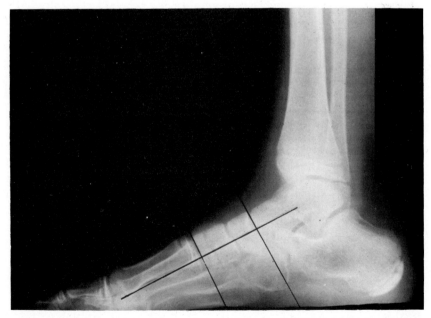

Figure 2. Roentgenographic appearance of foot in standing position in a 10 year old. The talonavicular and naviculocuneiform joints are normally aligned yet the foot is pronated clinically.

the embryo is approximately four weeks old and has at least 25 to 28 pairs of somites. They, however, do not contribute to the limb buds. Each limb bud grows in a proximodistal sequence: thigh, leg, foot; and within the foot: tarsus, metatarsus, phalanges. As the buds elongate, nerves and blood vessels grow rapidly into the limbs. Milaire[16] has showed that, although the skeletal blastemata appear in the depth of the limb, the tendons, muscles, and perichondrium arise by centripetal migration from the superficial mesenchyme.

At the beginning of the fifth week the foot anlage is oriented so that the future plantar surface faces the head. During the next two weeks the plantar surface rotates and comes to face more medially and more cephalad. At the end of the embryonic period, at approximately eight and one-half to nine weeks, the feet assume the "praying position," that is, the soles face medially and dorsally and the toes of one foot are generally in contact with the toes of the other. The foot is in line with the leg and is comparable to an equinus position. The talus and the calcaneus incline medially. Indications of the longitudinal arch of the foot are found. Böhm[3,4] has suggested that certain deformities of the foot develop at this embryonic stage because of failure of the foot to "rotate into pronation." A large part of this suggestion is conjecture rather than proved observation. Bardeen's[1] studies, although excellent, have not shed any additional light.

By the ninth postovulatory week, the various components of the foot have shapes, relationships, and anatomical arrangements similar to those found in the adult foot. It is during the fetal period that specific changes take place in the development of the talus. In the embryo the talus and the calcaneus are inclined medially so that the foot appears adducted. Before the end of the embryonic period lateral deviation begins to take place. During the fetal period the talus as a whole, which is on the medial side of the foot at first, shifts laterally to the longitudinal axis of the foot. In addition it gradually becomes relatively broader and higher; the neck is less medially directed along with an increased torsion of the talar head. These changes continue postnatally as well. Further careful studies not only of the normal fetal lower limbs but also of the abnormal ones are necessary in order to assess to what extent minimal deviations in the position of the talus in relation to the calcaneus and the navicular and the navicular to the medial cuneiform are responsible for the presence of flexible valgus type flatfoot deformity. Martinez and Gonzales[15] have emphasized that closely-graded, careful reconstruction, not only of the normal but more importantly of the abnormal feet, is absolutely necessary before any definite conclusions can be made.

## FUNCTIONAL PHYSIOLOGY

The properly balanced longitudinal arch depends upon the bony interrelationship of three joints—the talocalcaneal, the talonavicular, and the first naviculocuneiform. Loss of normal alignment of one or more of these joints resulting in plantar or valgus deviation of the midfoot or of the rearfoot will result in loss of the medial longitudinal arch.

It has been shown that muscle function is not responsible for maintenance of the longitudinal arch of the foot.[2,19]

The first line of support of the bony structures constituting the longitudinal arch is the ligaments. Basmajian and Bentzon[2] and earlier, Dudley Morton,[18] on the basis of various calculations, demonstrated that the static strain upon the ligaments required to sustain the normal or the flattened longitudinal arch is low in intensity and falls well within the capability of the ligaments. Therefore they concluded independently that: (1) The integrity of the arch is solely dependent upon the anatomical position and proper alignment of the articular surfaces of one bone in relation to the other. (2) The ligamentous function is solely one of holding the tarsal bones together. (3) The function of the muscles is to propel the foot and not to maintain the longitudinal arch, providing the muscles are of normal power. (4) Any loss of power of one group of muscles or of one particular muscle can result in various types of deformities of the foot.

Butte[5] was the first investigator in English literature who unequivocally stated:

The author believes that it (the tibialis anterior) has no arch elevating or supporting value for the following reasons: (1) It inverts or supinates the forefoot on the rearfoot producing one of the elements of flatfoot. (2) It elevates the first metatarsal head and the anterior limb of the medial longitudinal arch, directly opposing the action of the peroneus longus, and produces a lowering of the medial longitudinal arch. (3) In walking it contracts only during the swing phase of the step and during the instant of heel weight bearing as the advanced foot is put to the ground and the forefoot is lowered. As the weight moves forward to the forefoot, putting the greatest strain on the arch, the tibialis anterior is relaxed. (4) When it acts against a contracted gastrocnemius, or attempts to dorsiflex the foot against superimposed weight, it throws a further strain on the longitudinal arch. Further, since each of the actions of the tibialis anterior produces one of the elements of flatfoot, the writer [Butte] believes that weakness or paralysis of this muscle alone, particularly in a growing foot, is an important factor in the production of an exaggerated arch or clawfoot, the mirror image of a flatfoot. (Fig. 3.)

## ROENTGENOGRAPHIC EVALUATION

In standing roentgenograms of the normal foot taken after the age of three, the line bisecting the talus (Fig. 4A) should cross the navicular at a right angle to a line drawn over the navicular proximal articular surface. When the line is projected forward, it should bisect the cuneiform at a right angle to a line drawn parallel to the distal surface of the medial cuneiform. When projected distally, it should extend to the plantar surface of the first metatarsal head. On proximal projection it should bisect the head of the talus and run parallel to the trabeculae of the head and neck of the talus. This line (extending from the talus to the plantar aspect of the first metatarsal head) can be a straight one or slightly angulated dorsally at the naviculocuneiform joint.

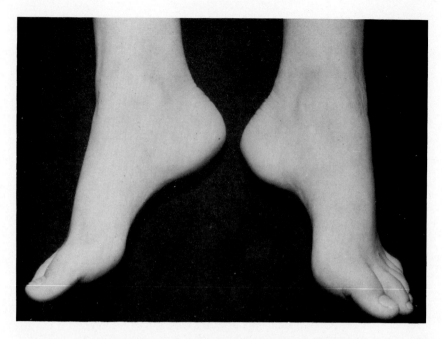

Figure 3. Feet of a nine year old girl who suffered an unrecognized laceration of the left tibialis anterior at age four at ankle joint level. Note normal right foot and cavus deformity of the left foot. There was no other muscle imbalance of the left foot.

In the standing anteroposterior view a line bisecting the neck of the talus (Fig. 4B) forms an angle of between 60 and 80 degrees with a line running parallel to the flattened portion of the distal articular surface of the navicular. This is the dorsoplantar talonavicular angle. An angle less than 60 degrees is considered abnormal. The medial deviation of the talus to the navicular is also contributory to valgus flatfoot deformity as is the sag of the naviculocuneiform joint with or without plantar flexion of the talus. Lack of recognition in the past may have been one of the factors that resulted in only approximately 60 per cent success in such procedures as advocated by Hoke,[10] Kidner,[9,11] Young,[20] Chambers,[7] and LeLievre,[12, 13] to name a few.

Valgus type flatfoot can be a result of plantar and/or valgus deviation of any one of the three components that constitute the longitudinal arch, namely the talocalcaneal, talonavicular, and medial naviculocuneiform joints. Flexible valgus flatfoot can also result from malalignment of only one of these joints, but more frequently results from loss of normal alignment of two of these components and in rare instances from malposition of all three (Fig. 5, A and B).

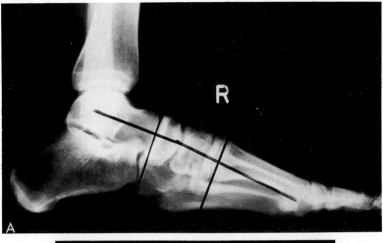

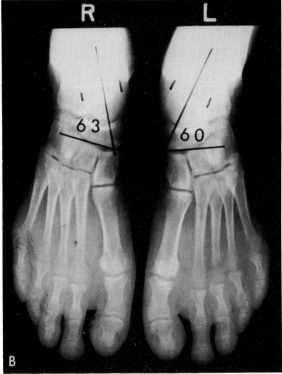

Figure 4.   *A*, Standing lateral roentgenogram of the normal foot. The line bisecting the neck and head of the talus bisects the navicular and the medial cuneiform parallel to the trabeculae of these three osseous structures. The line is angulated dorsally at the naviculocuneiform joint and extends to the plantar aspect of the first metatarsal head. A straight line is considered the lower limit of normal. *B*, Normal dorsoplantar talonavicular angle. Note that the line bisecting the neck and head of the talus forms an angle of between 60 and 80 degrees with a line drawn parallel to the distal articular surface of the navicular.

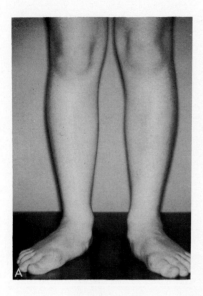

Figure 5. *A*, Bilateral, severe flatfeet resulting from malalignment of all three components that make up the longitudinal arch.

## CLINICAL APPEARANCE

PRONATED FOOT RESULTING FROM MEDIAL DEVIATION OF THE TALONAVICULAR JOINT. The foot appears flat in the standing anteroposterior view (Fig. 6*A*). However the longitudinal arch is normal when viewed from the medial standing position (Fig. 6*B*). This apparent flattening appears in the anteroposterior position because of the medial prominence of the head of the talus and the apparent eversion of the ankle joint. On true passive ankle extension (extension through the ankle joint with the subtalar joint locked) the foot can be brought up to a right angle position in relation to the leg. There is no contracture of the triceps surae or "shortening of the tendo calcaneus." On relative passive extension (extension of the foot with the subtalar joint unlocked) the foot can be extended 10 to 15 degrees beyond the neutral position.

In the standing roentgenograms (Fig. 7*A*) this eversion is a result of medial deviation of the talus in relation to the navicular with resulting talonavicular sag. In the standing lateral view (Fig. 7*B*) of the foot the alignment is normal.

VALGUS FOOT RESULTING FROM SAG OF THE NAVICULOCUNEIFORM JOINT. This is the most common type of flexible flatfoot deformity. The foot is flat in appearance (Fig. 8, *A* and *B*) in both the anteroposterior and medial standing positions with heel valgus (Fig. 8*C*). There is little evidence of a longitudinal arch. In approximately 10 to 15 per cent of these feet, when tested with true passive extension, there is contracture of the triceps surae or short tendo calcaneus. Relative passive extension is greater than the 10 degrees found in the normal foot.

On examination of the standing roentgenograms, there is plantar

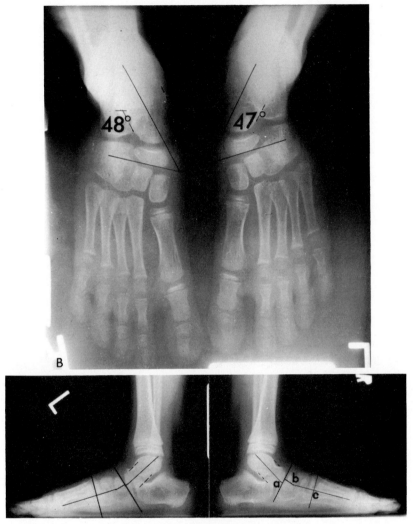

Figure 5 (*Continued*). *B*, Standing roentgenograms of the same feet. Note that in the anteroposterior view the dorsoplantar talonavicular angle is diminished and measures 48 degrees in the right foot and 47 degrees in the left. In the lateral standing views there is moderate plantar flexion of the talus (*a*) as well as plantar sag at the talonavicular joint (*b*). The tarsometatarsal joint (*c*) is normal and the line drawn at right angles to this articulation projects forward touching the plantar aspect of the first metatarsal head.

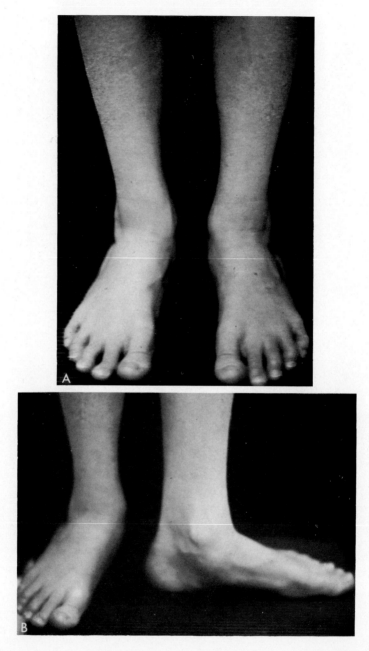

Figure 6.  *A*, In the anteroposterior view the feet appear to be moderately pronated. *B*, The same feet, when viewed from the medial aspect, present no evidence of pronation.

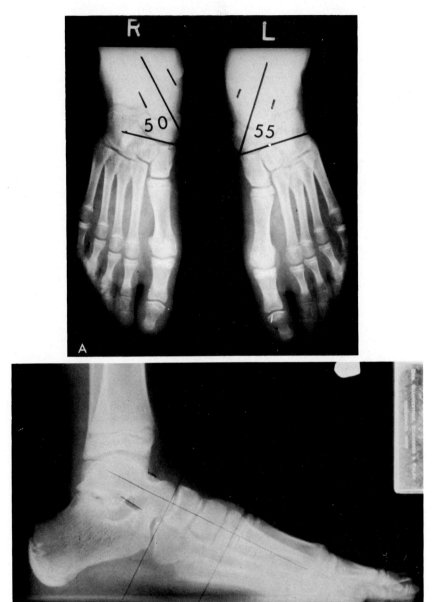

Figure 7. *A*, Standing anteroposterior roentgenographic evidence of medial deviation of the talus with resultant diminution of the dorsoplantar talonavicular angle. *B*, Lateral standing view of the same foot. Note normal alignment of the other two components of the longitudinal arch.

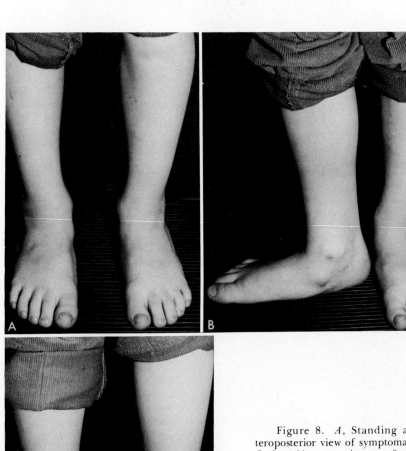

Figure 8. *A*, Standing anteroposterior view of symptomatic flatfeet. Note prominence of medial malleolus and absence of the longitudinal arch. *B*, Medial standing view. There is complete loss of the longitudinal arch. *C*, Note valgus position of heels.

sag of the naviculocuneiform joint (Fig. 9*A*). There may or may not be an appreciable diminution of the dorsoplantar talonavicular angle (Fig. 9*B*).

Valgus Foot Resulting from Plantar Flexion of the Talus.   In this type of flatfoot the talus is plantar flexed and deviated

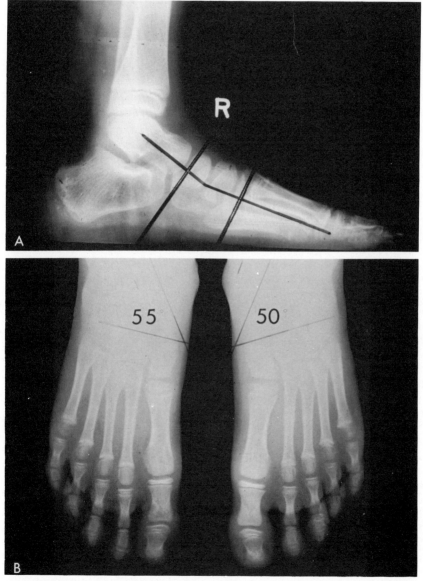

Figure 9.   *A*, Standing lateral roentgenogram. Note plantar angulation of the naviculocuneiform joint. *B*, Standing anteroposterior view. the dorsoplantar talonavicular angle is diminished in size.

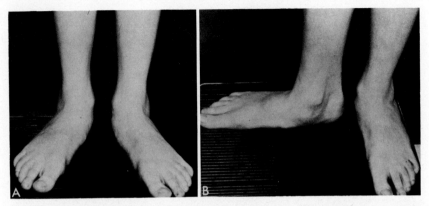

Figure 10. *A*, Standing anteroposterior view of flatfeet caused by plantar flexion of the talus. Note medial soft tissue prominence just below the malleolus due to plantar medial deviation of talar head. *B*, Medial view of the right foot. Note complete absence of the longitudinal arch. The heel is in valgus position producing an apparent deviation of the hindpart of the foot on the forepart of the foot.

medially in relationship to the calcaneus and the navicular. The head of the talus is prominent and palpable when the patient is standing (Fig. 10*A*). There is complete absence of the longitudinal arch (Fig. 10*B*). The heel is in valgus position and there is a deviation of the hindpart of the foot in the forepart of the foot. This is due to the marked sag at the talonavicular joint in the dorsoplantar plane.

The appearance of the standing roentgenograms in this type of foot is typical. The talus is plantar flexed in the lateral standing view (Fig. 10 *C*) with plantar deviation of the bisecting line between the talus and the navicular. In the standing anteroposterior view there is medial deviation of the talus in relation to the navicular (Fig. 10*D*) with diminution of the dorsoplantar talonavicular angle.

Severe valgus flatfoot of this type can at times be easily confused both clinically as well as roentgenographically with congenital rigid flatfoot (Fig. 11). However in congenital rigid flatfoot there is invariably contracture of the triceps surae. The heel is in neutral position when viewed from the posterior aspect. The valgus deviation of the forepart and midpart of the foot is the result of dorsolateral dislocation of the talonavicular joint. In the plantar flexed talus type of flatfoot, contracture of the triceps surae seldom occurs. The foot is flexible and the talus can be manipulated into normal position. The congenital rigid flatfoot is held in rigid valgus and cannot be easily corrected to neutral position.

Roentgenographically, in flexible valgus flatfoot of this type, the talus is plantar flexed, but not in the vertical position. In congenital rigid flatfoot it is almost at a right angle to the calcaneus. In flexible valgus flatfoot the os calcis is not in equinus as in congenital rigid flatfoot. The neck of the talus is not short as in the congenital rigid foot and the head of the talus is only slightly flattened (Fig. 12, *A* and *B*).

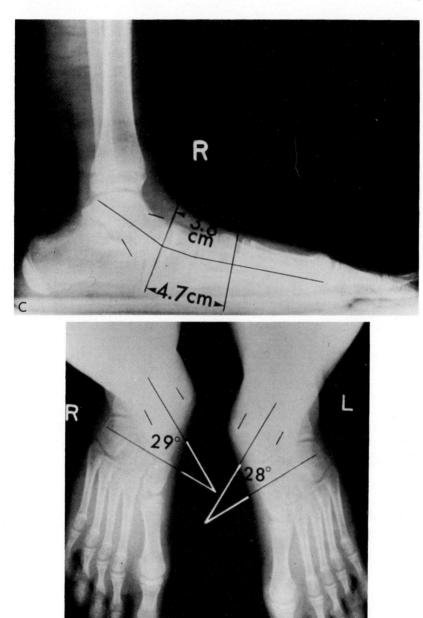

Figure 10 (*Continued*). *C*, Lateral standing view. The loss of alignment is between the talus and the navicular principally resulting from plantar flexion of the talus. There may or may not be a minimal sag of the naviculocuneiform joint. *D*, Anteroposterior standing roentgenogram. Note marked diminution of the dorsoplantar talonavicular angle. Medial deviation of the head of the talus in relation to the navicular is a constant finding in the flatfoot deformity caused by plantar flexion of the talus.

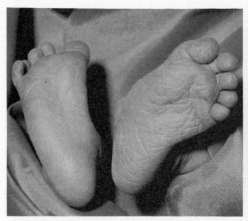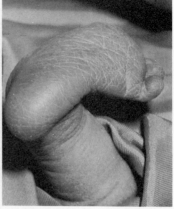

Figure 11.  Left congenital rigid flatfoot. Note valgus deviation of the distal two-thirds of the forefoot in relation to the hindpart. This is a result of dorsolateral subluxation of the navicular on the talus with occasional disalignment of the calcaneal cuboid joint as well.

## MATERIAL AND METHODS

All patients were treated conservatively for a period of from two to 10 years. The conservative measures consisted of corrective shoes or Whitman arch supports. Only 1 per cent of the patients seen for flexible valgus flatfoot have required surgical correction. In all others conservative therapy has yielded fair to good results. Some feet did not correct adequately with conservative means. However since they were completely asymptomatic and the parents' feet were equally as flat and still asymptomatic, surgery was not recommended. The majority of patients on whom surgery was performed did not complain of pain in their feet as long as the corrective measures were maintained. However when these were discontinued, the patient developed foot pain or unwillingness to walk because of general fatigue, clumsiness in gait, so-called "growing pains," fatigue when participating in sports, and other symptoms confined to the low back and lower extremity areas indicative of foot dysfunction. In such patients surgery was recommended. There was a small group of patients whose feet were asymptomatic but flat after all support was removed. Corrective surgery was recommended in such patients because one of the parents had similar feet that were disablingly painful, even though the feet were asymptomatic during youth. It was felt that the youngster's feet would eventually become symptomatic. This was discussed with the parents; the operative procedure was presented to them and the decision was left to them. Few youngsters' feet were corrected for cosmetic reasons only.

There is a familial tendency toward flatfeet (Fig. 13). This hereditary tendency may be either paternal, maternal, or both. There was no

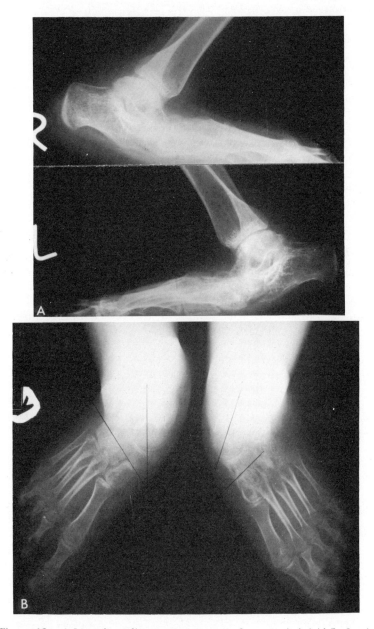

Figure 12. *A*, Lateral standing roentgenograms of a congenital rigid flatfoot in a 14 year old patient. Note equinus position of the calcaneus and vertical position of the talus. The navicular is displaced dorsally and laterally in relation to the talus. *B*, Standing anteroposterior roentgenogram of congenital rigid flatfeet. The dorsoplantar talonavicular angle measures 30 degrees on the right and 29 degrees on the left.

statistical significance in the preponderance of the appearance of flatfeet in the male parent as compared with the female parent. A number of the youngsters were brought for therapy because the feet, although apparently asymptomatic, were flat in appearance. After corrective measures had been prescribed, these children suddenly realized that they had had sore feet all along and that their feet were now asymptomatic for the first time in their young lives.

The ideal age for the surgical correction of flexible flatfeet in the adolescent is between the ages of 10 and 12 in the female and 12 and 14 in the male. By allowing an additional one and one-half to two years' growth of the foot, any readjustment of the articular surfaces as a result of the surgery can be easily effected. In the older patient (after age 14) one was less likely to obtain a good result. Therefore this procedure is not recommended for patients beyond the age of 14 except in carefully selected cases. In this series, three patients have been adults; all were females. The oldest was 41 years of age at the time of surgery (Fig. 14A). Each had severe disability consisting of disabling foot, leg, and back pain. Each had exhausted every means of conservative therapy, including "space shoes," prior to surgery. On examination all three patients' feet were extremely flexible and the feet could be manipulated into the normal position. Roentgenographically the findings were evident. There was naviculocuneiform sag in the lateral standing views and diminution of the dorsoplantar talonavicular angle in the anteroposterior view (Fig. 14, B to D). All three patients experienced moderate to good relief with the use of Whitman plates for a short period of time. All three were willing to accept the risk of surgery (Fig. 15, A and B). Figure 16 illustrates the postoperative appearance of one of these patients. The patients were improved but not totally asymptomatic. Each complained of some stiffness and soreness in the feet that was tolerable even after a day of heavy house cleaning.

The maximal follow-up for surgery was 24 years and the minimal follow-up was 4 years; the average is 7.5 years. The patient who underwent surgery 24 years ago is the mother of three children. Her feet are totally asymptomatic and well balanced. Several male patients have served in the Armed Forces and one was accepted in one of the Service schools and military life.

The method of rating results was the four point system with four points for excellent, three for very good, two for good, one for fair and zero for poor in four categories: cosmetic appearance, roentgenographic appearance, subjective symptomatology, and function (range of motion as compared to the normal foot). A total of 16 points was rated as excellent, 15 as very good, 14 as good, 13 as fair, and 12 or less as poor. Thus a fair cosmetic appearance with moderate limitation of motion would automatically rate as 12 points or less and be considered a poor foot in spite of the fact that both roentgenographically subjectively the foot might be rated as excellent. A patient, therefore, might be satisfied with his feet in that they were asymptomatic and not be concerned about the moderate loss of tarsal motion and fair cosmetic appearance yet these feet would be rated as a poor result. The majority of patients were evaluated independently by two examiners.

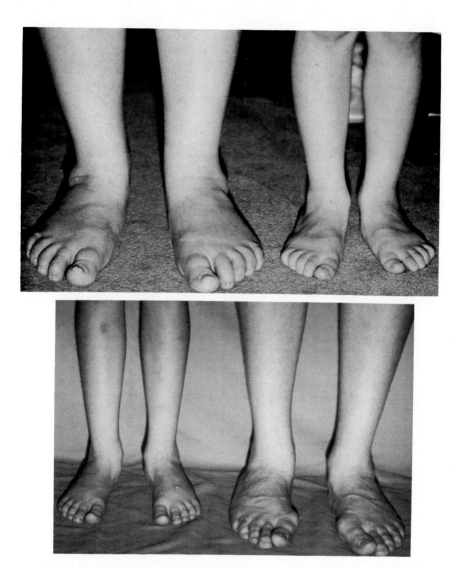

Figure 13. Familial diathesis of flatfeet. Both illustrations are mother and daughter combinations. Note the striking resemblance in the structure and appearance of each of these two pairs of feet.

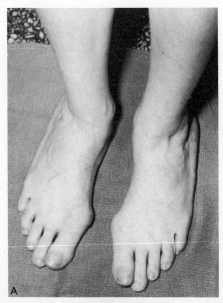

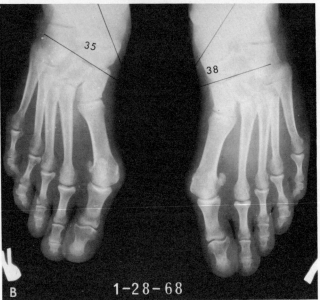

Figure 14.  *A*, Severely symptomatic flatfeet in a 41 year old adult. Note the valgus position of the entire foot as well as the heel bilaterally. *B*, Preoperative appearance of both feet in the standing position. Observe medial deviation of the talar head with resultant diminution of the dorsoplantar talonavicular angle to 35 degrees in the right foot and 38 degrees in the left foot. The normal angle is between 60 to 80 degrees.

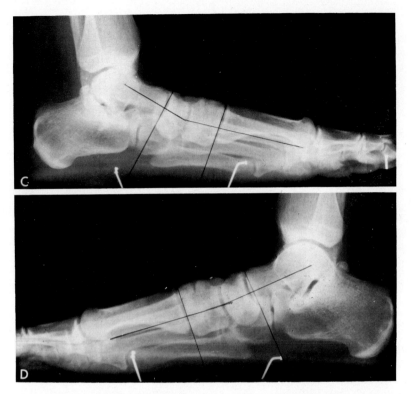

Figure 14 (*Continued*). *C*, Lateral standing roentgenogram of right foot. There is a marked sag plantarly at the naviculocuneiform joint. The talonavicular joint relationship is normal in appearance in the lateral standing view. *D*, The naviculocuneiform sag is not as severe in the left foot.

## DISCUSSION

The operative procedure found to be best suited for the correction of adolescent flexible valgus flatfoot resulting from a sag of the naviculocuneiform joint with or without medial sag of the talonavicular joint is the following modification of the Miller procedure. Under no circumstances should this operation be used to correct the flexible valgus flatfoot deformity resulting from plantar flexion of the talus. The ideal procedure for this type of valgus flatfoot is the Grice[8] operation, in conjunction with transplantation of the tibialis anterior under the navicular to correct the medial deviation of the talus on the navicular.

## OPERATIVE PROCEDURE

This operation is a combination of some elements of the Miller[17] operation and some of the more desirable features of other operations

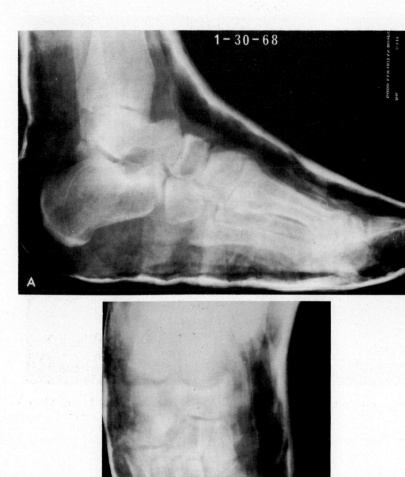

Figure 15. *A*, Immediate postoperative roentgenographic appearance of the right foot in the lateral view. The naviculocuneiform sag has been corrected. *B*, Anteroposterior roentgenographic view of the same foot. Note that the dorsoplantar talonavicular angle is now well corrected.

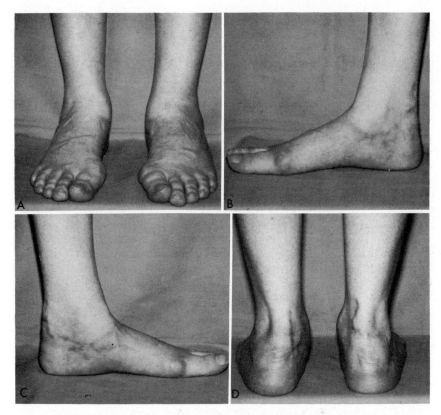

Figure 16. *A*, Appearance of feet 18 months after surgical correction. Except for slight stiffness and some swelling of the feet at the ankle joint level, the feet are asymptomatic and well balanced (compare with Figure 14*A*). *B* and *C*, Standing medial view of right and left foot. Observe the presence of the longitudinal arch in both feet. *D*, Posterior standing view. The right heel is in very minimal valgus position while the left is in neutral position.

such as the Kidner,[11] the Durham,[6] and the Lowman.[14] In addition to the development of the osteoperiosteal graft and arthrodesis of the naviculocuneiform joint, the tibialis anterior and posterior tendons are transplanted to the plantar aspect of the navicular. Transplantation of the tibialis posterior is carried out because the author has observed for the past 15 years a rather common finding in this type of valgus flatfoot, namely, that of the insertion of the tibialis posterior on the medial surface. Although repetitious, it should be reemphasized that the ideal ages for this operation are between 10 and 12 in the female and 12 and 14 in the male. When this operation has been performed at an earlier age than recommended, varus deformity distal to the naviculocuneiform arthrodesis has developed as the child has grown (Fig. 17).

The successive steps of the operative procedure follow. Under tourniquet control, a slightly curved incision is made along the medial surface of the foot beginning just posterior to the medial malleolus, extending forward to the navicular tubercle and then curving distally to the midshaft of the first metatarsal (Fig. 18). An inadequate incision will inevitably result in inability to correct the foot properly. The abductor hallucis is then carefully reflected from the medial and plantar surfaces of the cuneiform, navicular, and the spring ligament.

Posteriorly the common flexor digitorum longus tendon is identified with the medial branch of the posterior tibial nerve. The tibialis posterior tendon sheath should be split from the level of the medial malleolus to the navicular tubercle. The tendon should be detached from the tubercle with a moderate amount of the tendon covering over the navicular tubercle. This particular step in the detachment of the tibialis posterior tendon is important as will be demonstrated later. A 2-0 chromic catgut suture is passed through the tendon for the purpose of identification and traction (Fig. 19).

The tibialis anterior tendon is identified, freed from its tendon sheath from the inferior extensor retinaculum to the first tarsometatarsal joint, and is divided. An identifying 2-0 chromic catgut suture is passed through the tendon. Two parallel incisions 1.5 cm in width are made from the metatarsocuneiform joint to the talar neck at the sustentaculum tali. The capsular and ligamentous structures are incised down to the underlying bone. Care should be exercised to avoid cutting the tendon

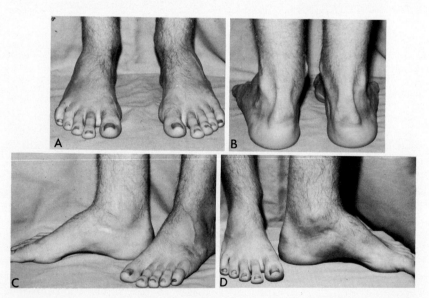

Figure 17. *A* and *B*, Standing anteroposterior and rear views of feet that were corrected surgically at the age of nine instead of age 12. Note slight varus of each forefoot that is better demonstrated in the posterior view. *C* and *D*, Standing medial view of same feet. Note the cavus deformity that has developed, particularly in the right foot.

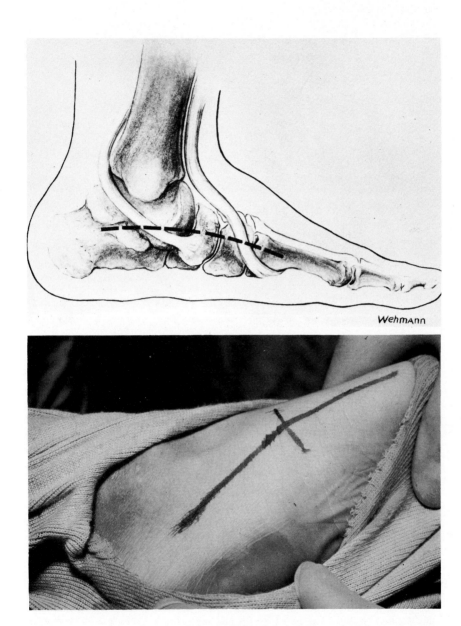

Figure 18.  Skin incision begins just behind the posterior edge of the medial malleolus and curves slightly dorsally to the junction of the proximal one-third and distal two-thirds of the first metatarsal shaft. A short incision will result in inability to correct the foot properly.

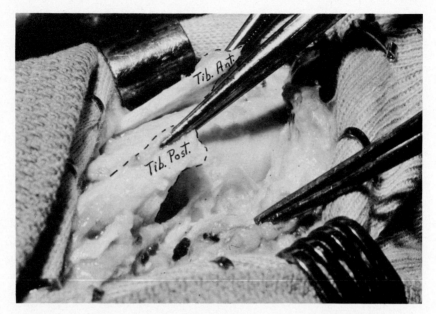

Figure 19.   The tibialis anterior and posterior tendons have been detached.

of the flexor digitorium longus or the medial plantar branch of the tibial nerve that lies just posterior to the tendon. The capsule of the first metatarsocuneiform joint is incised between the two parallel cuts. With a thin sharp osteotome an osseoligamentous flap is raised between the two parallel incisions beginning at the distal end of the medial cuneiform. A thin layer of the cortex of the cuneiform as well as of the navicular tubercle are removed along with the ligamentous structures covering the area of these two bones. The ligamentous structures over these two segments are quite thin and care must be exercised in raising the flap over these bones lest the osseoligamentous flap be torn. The spring ligament is dissected free to the level of the sustentaculum tali. As it is lifted back, the medial surface of the head and neck of the talus is exposed as well as the medial edge of the talocalcaneal joint (Fig. 20).

The ligamentous and capsular structures are dissected from the dorsal and plantar surfaces of the navicular and the medial cuneiform. The cortex of the plantar surface of the navicular is roughened to form a new bed for the tibialis anterior and posterior tibial tendons.

In order to correct the naviculocuneiform sag it is necessary to remove a thin wedge of bone from the proximal surface of the medial cuneiform. The base of the wedge is located plantarward. This should not be more than 2 to 3 mm in width (Fig. 21). The apex of the wedge should consist of little else but the articular cartilage. A thin sharp osteotome is mandatory. The apposing navicular articular surface is then denuded of articular cartilage, exposing the underlying cortex. The forefoot is pronated and plantar flexed to make certain that the correc-

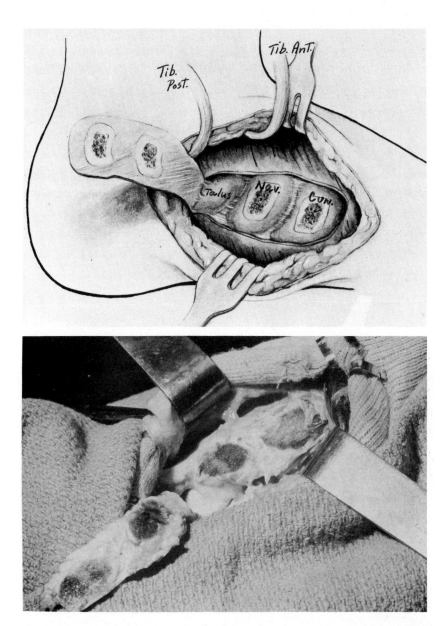

Figure 20. The osteoperiosteal graft has been detached and dissected free to the sustentaculum tali.

tion is adequate and that there is good apposition of the bone surfaces. Then a drill hole 5/16 inch in diameter is made in the cuneiform beginning on the plantar surface just proximal to the distal articular edge of the medial cuneiform. It should extend proximally and dorsally to the denuded articular surface just below the dorsal cortex. A second drill hole is made in the navicular from its plantar surface extending dorsally and distally, the drill exiting at the midportion of the denuded articular

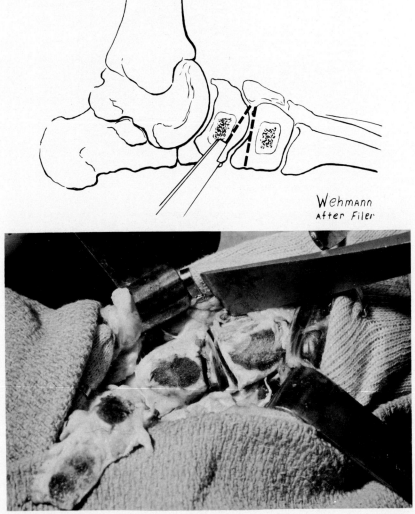

Wehmann
After Filer

Figure 21.   Only the articular cartilage and a minimal amount of cortex are resected from the navicular. The wedge of bone is removed from the medial cuneiform with the base of the wedge on the plantar surface. Care must be exercised lest too large a wedge is excised.

surface of the navicular. Care must be exercised in preparing these suture openings to ensure an adequate amount of cortex in both bones so that the suture does not tear out of the underlying cancellous bone when the ligature is passed through and tied. A double 2 chromic catgut suture is passed from the plantar surface of the navicular through the proximal superior opening of the cuneiform and out the plantar surface of this latter structure (Fig. 22). While the forefoot is held in the desired corrected position, the assistant ties the suture.

The foot is then held in the maximally corrected position, particularly as it applies to the talonavicular joint, and the osseoligamentous flap is pulled taut with the use of a Kocher clamp to cover the surfaces of the navicular and cuneiform bones. The flap should present a bowstring effect since an arch has already been constructed on the plantar medial aspect of the midtarsal portion of the foot. With the flap held in this position, a 0 chromic catgut suture on as fine a small cutting needle as will accommodate this suture is passed through the capsular structures attached to the base of the first metatarsal, then through the flap proximal to the cuneiform cortex (Fig. 23). The foot is held in the adducted position and the suture is tied securely. Two additional sutures are applied. The redundant portion of the flap is then sectioned (Fig. 24). The foot can now be released by the assistant. It will be observed that the correction is automatically maintained and that the flap is bowstrung on the plantar medial aspect of the tarsal region of the foot.

A second drill hole 7/64 inch in diameter is made in the navicular for the tibialis anterior and posterior tendons. The plantar surface of the navicular should be completely denuded of soft tissues and the cortex roughened. A 2 chromic catgut suture is passed in a figure 8 fashion through both tendon ends. The two suture ends are threaded into the needle and pulled through the bone. The two tendons are pulled over the flap and are guided to the plantar surface of the navicular. As the suture is pulled into the navicular the foot goes into slight varus. A Kocher clamp should be used to hold the tendons to the plantar surface of the navicular as the suture is tied. Additional sutures are then applied along the superior and inferior edges of the osteoperiosteal flap and the adjoining capsular structures until the closure is complete (Fig. 24). One or two sutures are applied through the tendons and the underlying spring ligament. The tendon sheath of the tibialis posterior should be repaired.

A hemovac unit is inserted with the exit of the tube in the distal calf. Following careful closure of the subcutaneous tissues, the skin should be closed with a subcuticular wire suture.

If there is evidence of a short tendocalcaneus prior to the anticipated corrective surgery, lengthening of the tendon should be performed first.

The application of the postoperative cast is of paramount importance. *It must be applied by the surgeon.* Immobilization in overcorrection is undesirable. The cast should be applied to *hold* the foot in the corrected position and should not be applied with the idea that it will correct the foot. Correction is performed surgically. The cast should be well molded about the corrected longitudinal arch and should be applied snugly (Fig.

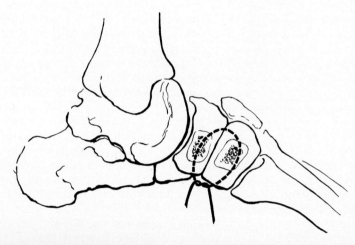

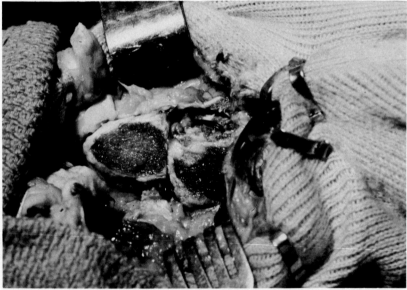

Figure 22.    Suture in situ. A No. 2 double chromic catgut suture is applied through the previously prepared drill holes, the defect closed by a adducting and pronating the forefoot. The suture must be tied on the plantar surface.

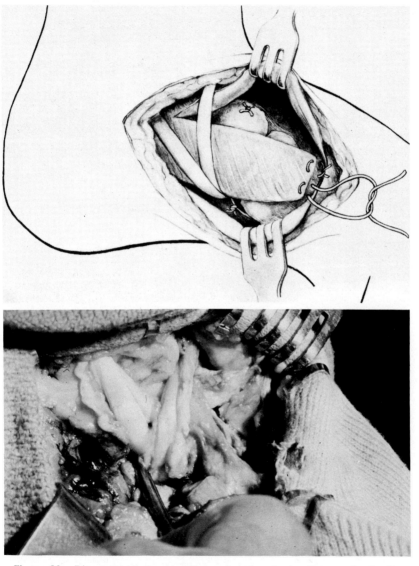

Figure 23. Diagrammatic sketch of flap and tendons in situ. See text for details.

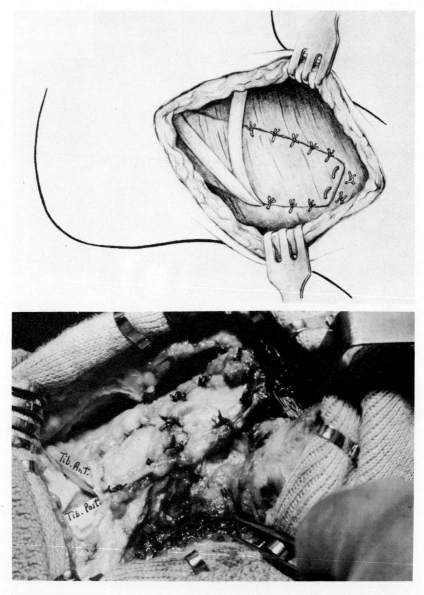

Figure 24. Reattachment of the osteoperiosteal graft and tendons completed.

25). Too much sheet wadding is undesirable. One should not anticipate changing the cast two weeks after surgery for a more snugly fitting one. Only very occasionally will this be necessary. If a change is required, it should be carried out under general anesthesia.

The cast is applied in sections. First, using four inch wide rolls of extra fast plaster of Paris, the lower one-fourth of the leg, the ankle, and the foot to the level of the midmetatarsal level is wrapped. The foot should be held from the toes in the neutral position with the knee held in 90 degrees of flexion. The plaster roll should be applied from outside toward the inside so that the minimal varus of the heel is not disturbed. It should be wrapped snugly about the newly formed longitudinal arch. After the application of one or two rolls, the plaster is molded firmly under the longitudinal arch and around the heel. The tourniquet is then released. After this portion of the cast has set, the remaining portion of the foot is wrapped with the forefoot held in a position of maximal pronation. The forepart of the foot is maintained in pronation and molded on the plantar surface. The remainder of the leg is incorporated in the cast up to the level of the tibial tubercle. The cast should then be well reinforced with additional plaster of Paris splints and rolls of plaster. The toes should be held parallel to each other in the cast.

## POSTOPERATIVE CARE

The foot should be elevated on two pillows with ice bags applied for the first 48 hours. Sedation should be quite liberal since the pain is quite intense. The usual child's dose according to weight and age is insufficient and it is neccssary to use adult doses for the first 36 to 48 hours.

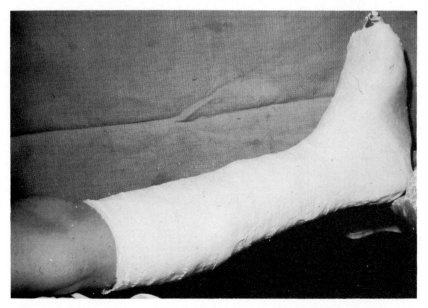

Figure 25. Completed cast. Note molding of cast under medial longitudinal arch.

The hemovac unit is removed on the third postoperative day. Postoperative roentgenograms in the anteroposterior and lateral views should be procured 24 hours following surgery to ascertain the position of the talonavicular and the naviculocuneiform joints respectively. The patient is permitted to become ambulatory five to seven days following surgery. No weight bearing is permitted on the corrected foot. One week after this, one can correct the opposite foot if he so desires. Immobilization is maintained for a minimum of eight weeks.

The surgeon should forewarn the parents that the feet will appear to be overcorrected when the restrictive dressings are removed. They should be reassured that this apparent overcorrection will disappear within 14 to 21 days after active walking is initiated. Roentgenograms are procured upon removal of the casts to ascertain the fusion of the naviculocuneiform joint. Occasionally, the fusion may appear to be weak but this is of no immediate consequence. If there is roentgenographic evidence of nonunion, however, a walking cast should be applied for another four weeks. If a nonunion should persist after this 12 week period, disregard it. In only one patient in this series has it been necessary to refuse an ununited naviculocuneiform joint because of pain. The remaining feet in which nonunion was present have remained symptom-free in spite of the lack of fusion. In one recent patient, fracture of the fusion site occurred eight months after surgery. The foot was painful for approximately six months. No additional immobilization of the foot was carried out. The foot gradually became asymptomatic as the fusion area gradually solidified.

The patient should be fitted with a new pair of rigid shanked, oxford type shoes as soon as the casts are removed. Ambulation with crutches under the supervision of a physical therapist is instituted. The patient is instructed in the proper heel-toe gait from the beginning. He should not be permitted to walk with the previously accustomed flatfoot gait. Exercises to strengthen the extensors as well as the triceps surae group of muscles are prescribed.

At first the youngster tends to walk on the lateral aspect of each foot and does not use his toes in proper take-off. The parents should be reassured that this poor gait will gradually disappear spontaneously as the patient learns to walk properly. The youngster is encouraged to discard crutches as soon as possible. The majority of patients discard crutches by the second week. Instruction in gait training should be continued until the patient walks with a normal pattern. No arch supports are fitted in the shoes. All athletic activities are prohibited during the first six postoperative months. The youngsters can wear any type of shoe they wish three months after surgery, providing the style is not extreme.

## The "Don'ts" of the Operation

Do not use staples to maintain the naviculocuneiform correction. In each instance in which they have been used, it was necessary to remove them. Do not hesitate to split the cast and sheet wadding to relieve circulatory impairment, but do not remove the foot from the posterior two-thirds of the cast. If infection is suspected, window the cast to expose the entire incision, remove the skin sutures to permit drainage, and treat the infection parenterally. *Above all, the entire cast should not be removed.*

One should not attempt to correct both feet at the same sitting. The operating time will average one and one-half hours.

Do not insert any type of arch support in the shoes postoperatively. The youngster must not be permitted to resume his flatfooted gait after surgery. Demonstrate both to the patient and the parents the proper method of heel-toe walking. If one does not take the time to do so, the youngster will walk clumsily for months. Rarely, a patient will develop spasm of the peroneal muscles because of the lack of instruction in proper walking. Do not permit such spasm to persist. Manipulate the foot gently under general anesthesia and immobilize it in a walking cast for six weeks. Upon removal of the cast, make certain that the youngster receives proper gait training as well as foot exercises to obviate the recurrence of this problem.

The minimal period of follow-up is 24 months after surgical correction. The patient should be checked bi-weekly for six weeks, once monthly for six months, and then every six months. Check-up roentgenograms should be procured 3, 6, 12, 18 and 24 months after surgical correction.

## FOLLOW-UP STUDY

A total number of 120 patients have undergone surgical correction. Ten patients have been lost to follow-up. In 22 patients the records were incomplete because the patient failed to return for examination in spite of being reminded. In eight of the patients included in the study, other orthopedists were kind enough to complete the follow-up examination including photographs and roentgenograms. Several of the male patients in this age group have been on active service with the Armed Forces. Of the patients who were evaluated in our office at least 75 per cent were examined by two orthopedic surgeons. A total of 146 feet have been corrected surgically in 88 patients.

The analysis will be made on the number of feet and not on the number of patients since in several patients one foot would be rated as excellent and the other foot as very good, fair, or poor as the case may be.

A four point system of rating was established. On this four point system an excellent cosmetic rating was given to the foot that was perfectly normal in appearance. A mild valgus of the heel or a minimal varus would reduce the rating to three points. If the correction had resulted in the development of a mild cavus, the foot was given a two point rating; a varus of the midfoot was given a one point rating; and if the foot were so overcorrected as to constitute a deformity, the rating was zero and the foot was judged to be a poor result. On the other hand, if there was slight pronation of the foot a two point rating was given. If the foot still appeared pronated but not completely flat, the rating was zero or considered to be poor result. Similarly normal tarsal motion was rated four, minimal loss of inversion of the foot was rated three, mild to moderate loss was rated two, and complete loss of motion was rated as zero or failure.

Roentgenographically a normal appearing foot was given a four point rating. If there was insufficient correction of the

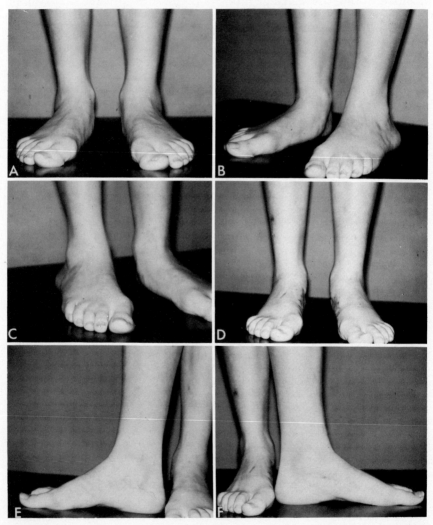

Figure 26. *A*, Standing views in the anteroposterior position. Note the prominence of the medial aspect of each foot and complete absence of the longitudinal arch. *B* and *C*, Standing side views. Note valgus of heels and absence of medial and lateral longitudinal arches. *D*, Postoperative appearance of same feet 13 months later. The eversion has been corrected. *E* and *F*, Medial views of right and left foot. Note the well defined longitudinal arch. The feet are normal in appearance.

naviculocuneiform joint or the dorsoplantar talonavicular angle, a three point rating was given. When both components were incompletely corrected the rating was two. A nonunion of the naviculocuneiform joint was rated two even though the nonunion was asymptomatic. In none of the feet was the rating below two roentgenographically.

From a subjective standpoint asymptomatic feet were rated four; minimal discomfort after a full day's activity three; aching of the feet when standing for any length of time, two; painful feet at the end of the day's work, one; and complete recurrence of the symptoms, zero.

Under the series of rather strict evaluation, 79 feet received 16 points—excellent; 32 feet received 15 points—very good; 16 feet received 14 points—good; 10 feet received 13 points—fair; and nine feet received 12 points or less—poor. Thus 127 of the 146 feet were rated from excellent to good (Fig. 26). Of the seven feet rated only as fair, there was nonunion of the naviculocuneiform joint arthrodesis in two. In two feet the result was considered to be only fair because in each case the patient complained of sufficient pain after a day's work to cause the patient to be only partially pleased with the operation. Metatarsalgia and callus formation under the second and third metatarsal heads resulting in the use of metatarsal pads on occasion was another reason for a fair rating in two feet. In the seventh foot of this group the reason for the

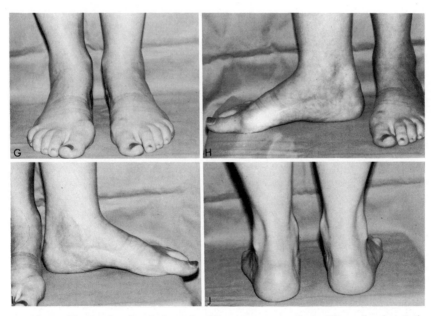

Figure 26 (*Continued*). *G*, Same feet 15 years postoperatively. The patient is now the mother of two children. Her feet are asymptomatic. *H* and *I*, Medial view of right and left foot 15 years after surgical correction. Note the well developed, normal-appearing arch. *J*, Note the well balanced heels. There is no valgus as seen in the preoperative illustrations in *B* and *C*.

fair rating, in spite of no complaints on the part of the patient, was the limitation of tarsal motion to approximately half the normal range.

The failures occurred during early years of experience. There have been no poor results during the past 15 years that this surgical procedure has been performed. In one patient, cavovarus deformity developed because the patient's feet had been corrected at the age of nine (Fig. 17). In another patient a pressure area from the cast developed requiring a skin graft to the lateral malleolus. One child developed an infection and slough of the incision on both feet. After several weeks of hospitalization during which debridement of the incision was necessary, the wounds closed. Secondary plastic surgery consisting of application of pedicle flaps was necessary. The patient ambulates normally and has no complaints referable to her feet as far as function is concerned. The range of motion in each foot is minimally limited, but the cosmetic result is considered to be very poor. In one patient the result was considered to be poor because the feet were not symmetrically corrected. A two team approach was used resulting in the right foot being balanced and cosmetically excellent but the left foot was not as well corrected from a cosmetic standpoint. This produced a rather incongruous effect when the two feet were observed. It is on the basis of this case that the authors recommend that both feet be corrected by the same surgeon.

## CONCLUSIONS

This operation is not a panacea. It is indicated in flatfeet in which the deformity is the result of a plantar sag of the naviculocuneiform joint, a medial sag of the talonavicular joint, or a combination of the two. The author recommends that this operative procedure be carried out principally on symptomatic flatfeet. On the other hand, should the parents wish that the youngster's feet be corrected for cosmetic purposes only, this procedure can be performed providing the child's feet are flat roentgenographically as well as clinically because of the above-mentioned disalignment, and providing the parents have been advised of the possible complications that may ensue with the performance of such a surgical procedure. The maximal follow-up is 24 years and the minimal follow-up four years. Fifty-four per cent of the feet were considered to show excellent results, 22 per cent were evaluated as very good, and 11 per cent as good. Thus, 87 per cent of the corrected feet carefully studied were considered to have good to excellent results. The results in seven per cent were considered to be fair and in six per cent to be poor. The author does not claim any originality in this procedure. He has simply combined some of the more desirable features of the various operations described in the past. With careful attention to details and meticulous surgical technique the results of this procedure can be most satisfying to both the patient and the orthopedist.

# REFERENCES

A complete bibliography, containing additional references to historical background material, is available from the author upon request.

1. Bardeen, C. R.: Studies of the development of the human skeleton. Am. J. Anat., 4:265-302, 1905.

2. Basmajian, J. R., and Bentzon, J. W.: An electromyographic study of certain muscles of the leg and foot in the standing position. Surg. Gynecol. Obstet., 98:662-666, 1954.

3. Böhm, M.: Der Foetal Fuss. Beitragzue Ehtstehung des Pes Planus, des Pes Valgus und des Pes Planovalgus. Ztschr. F. Orthop. Chir., 57: 1932.

4. Böhm, M.: The embryologic origin of clubfoot. J. Bone Joint Surg., 11:229-259, 1929.

5. Butte, F.: Naviculocuneiform arthrodesis for flatfoot. J. Bone Joint Surg., 19:496-502, 1937.

6. Caldwell, G. D.: Surgical correction of relaxed flatfoot by the Durham flatfoot plasty. Clin. Orthop., 2:221-226, 1953.

7. Chambers, E. F. S.: An operation for the correction of flexible flatfeet of adolescents. West. J. Surg. Obstet. Gynecol., 14:77-86, 1946.

8. Grice, D. S.: An extra-articular arthrodesis of the subtalar joint for the correction of paralytic flatfeet in children. J. Bone Joint Surg., 34A:927-940, 1952.

9. Hibbs, R. A.: Muscle bound feet. N. Y. Med. J., 100:797-799, 1914.

10. Hoke, M.: An operation for the correction of extremely relaxed flatfeet. J. Bone Joint Surg., 13:773-783, 1931.

11. Kidner, F. C.: The prehallux (accessory scaphoid) in relation to flatfoot. J. Bone Joint Surg., 11:831, 1929.

12. LeLièvre, J.: Pathologie du Pied. Edition 1. Paris, Masson et Cie., 1967, pp. 228-230. 230.

13. LeLièvre, J.: Current concepts and correction in the valgus foot. J. Clin. Orthop., 70:43-55, 1970.

14. Lowman, C. L.: An operative method for correction of certain forms of flatfoot. J.A.M.A., 81:1500-1502, 1923.

15. Martinez Cuadrado, G., and Gonzáles Santander, R.: Contribución al estudio de la formacion y desarrollo del esqueleto del miembro inferior de embriones y fetos humanos, con especial referencia a los huesos del tarso. An. Desarrollo, 14:45-53, 1967.

16. Milaire, J.: Etude morphologique et cytochimique du développement des membres chez la souris et chez la taupe. Arch. Biol. Liège, 74:129-317, 1963.

17. Miller, O. L.: A plastic foot operation. J. Bone Joint Surg., 9:84-91, 1927.

18. Morton, D. J.: Human Locomotion and Body Form. A Study of Gravity and Man. Baltimore, The Williams and Wilkins Co., 1952.

19. Sheffield, F. J., Gersten, J. W., and Mastetone, A. F.: Electromyographic study of the muscles of the foot in normal walking. Am. J. Phys. Med., 35:223-236, 1956.

20. Young, C. S.: Operative treatment of pes planus. Surg. Gynecol. Obstet., 68:1099-1101, 1939.

*Chapter 8*

# Total Ankle Replacement Arthroplasty

KENNETH C. SCHOLZ, M.D.*

Total ankle replacement arthroplasty has created a whole new dimension in the management of advanced arthritic destructive changes of the ankle joint. Prior to the advent of total replacement arthroplasty, fusion of the ankle joint has been the only effective surgical method to eliminate pain in a destroyed joint. Unfortunately, motion is also eliminated with joint arthrodesis which is not always desirable. Elimination of motion in one joint could create additional problems to contiguous joints as well. The need to maintain and not eliminate motion in a joint has been documented. It is becoming customary among orthopedic surgeons to treat joints destroyed by arthritis with prosthetic replacement when indicated. Hip and finger joint replacements are at the present widely used and knee replacements are rapidly gaining acceptance. Replacement of the ankle joint is an entirely new concept.

In evaluating any surgical procedure in the arthritic patient important consideration must be given to the restoration of motion and stability of the involved joint. However, we cannot lose sight of the fact that pain is usually the major indication for all reconstructive surgical procedures in the arthritic patient and that success or failure of any procedure will ultimately be judged by its ability to eliminate or reduce pain in addition to restoration of acceptable joint motion and stability.

If the arthritic joint is to be replaced with prosthetic components then additional factors must be considered:

1. *Design* that should allow minimal wear.
2. *Construction* from materials known to be acceptable in an intraarticular environment.
3. *Prosthetic stability.* Prosthetic components should provide intrinsic lateral and rotary stability between the units.
4. *Joint stability.* Prosthetic replacements should preserve ligamentous support of the ankle.
5. *Minimal sacrifice of bone* so that arthrodesis can still be carried out as a salvage procedure should it become indicated in the future.

---

* Associate Clinical Professor of Orthopedic Surgery, Texas Tech University School of Medicine. Lubbock, Texas; Staff, Highland Hospital and Methodist Hospital, Lubbock, Texas.

6. *Versatility* to allow for correction of existing deformities of the ankle such as varus, valgus, equinus, calcaneus, or a combination of these attitudes.

7. *Prosthetic ankle motion* should allow sufficient tibiopedal motion for gait with a shoe. Tibiopedal motion should include at least 10 degrees of dorsiflexion (extension) and 25 degrees of plantarflexion (flexion) or a total of approximately 35 degrees of foot and ankle motion. In this range of motion the joint surfaces are always sliding across each other. True tibiotalar "ankle" motion represents only a portion of the total tibiopedal motion reported as 35 degrees during ambulation. Generally weight bearing studies as viewed on single roentgenographic exposure and cineradiography studies show flexion and extension to be approximately equal but these studies do not imply the value in ambulation during a walking cycle. These ambulatory values, of course, would be much less than the maximal limit found in flexion and extension weight bearing studies demonstrated on single exposure roentgenograms or cineradiograms.

8. *Avoidance* of designs which do not afford intrinsic stability against medial and lateral stresses that could lead to excessive loading of the prosthesis, thereby increasing the problems of wear and loosening. Prosthetic wear is also influenced by a polyethylene device that faces "up" so that loose particles might have a tendency to collect and subsequently be ground into the articular surface of the component. Implants using intramedullary implantation or external devices such as screws for fixation should also be avoided.

## INDICATIONS AND CONTRAINDICATIONS FOR SURGERY

The procedure is indicated in patients with advanced arthritic changes of the ankle who have disabling pain and limited motion that have not responded to conservative management. No age limit has been established due to the fact that all had advanced arthritic changes and were considered candidates for tibiotalar arthrodesis. The primary aim is to alleviate pain and, secondarily, restore motion and provide stability.

The indications are the same as those to replace other joints with prosthetic devices: traumatic degenerative arthritis, osteoarthritis without antecedent history of trauma, rheumatoid arthritis, and failure of previous surgical procedures. Contraindications are similar to the restrictions of prosthetic replacement in other joints: previous joint sepsis, neuropathy, ligamentous instability of the ankle, and vascular insufficiency of the lower extremity.

## DESIGN AND PROSTHETIC CHARACTERISTICS

The advantages and disadvantages of metal on plastic versus metal on metal and the utilization of polymethymethacrylate are well documented and will not be discussed.[1, 3-6, 12, 13, 16-20] The talar component is constructed of chrome-cobalt-molybdenum alloy and the tibial component of ultra high molecular weight (UHMW) high density polyethylene. Both components are fixed with methyl methacrylate. Experimentally the final angular total contact model accepted was the design which imparted the greatest degree of intrinsic stability when the ankle is loaded during weight bearing ambulatory activities or while standing on various surfaces (Fig. 1). The resistance against varus, valgus, rotary, and other stresses is necessary to dissipate forces from the ankle distally to the subtalar joint as well as to the talonavicular joint and even proximally to the knee joint. If this intrinsic stability is not present especially in dorsiflexion as the talus tends to "lock into the ankle mortise" or when ambulating or standing on uneven surfaces such as up, down, or laterally on an incline plane then a "rolling or twisting" type of subluxation will occur. This would have a tendency to overstretch stabilizing ankle ligaments and concentrate forces over a small area of the prosthetic components. The expected result would be ankle pain caused by overstretched ligaments and accelerated wear of the prosthetic units or even a loosening effect of the prosthesis from the bone interface. The angular edge of the talar component is not sharp enough to increase wear or cause breakage of the tibial component because of the total contact design that evenly distributes a pressure load over the wide surface of the prosthesis. The prosthesis probably should not be utilized in active younger people where a subtalar arthrodesis is also necessary although this has not been established. The range of motion of the unit is approximately 70 degrees and closely approximates the radius of curvature found in normal tibiotalar joints.[21] The talar component is wider anteriorly and gently narrows posteriorly to simulate normal talar action during ankle motion. The ligamentous integrity of the ankle is left intact.

If the ankle is without ligamentous support the prosthetic replacement should not be contemplated. The more narrow, sloping surface is always medial and the wider surface is lateral. The nonarticular surface of the talar component has two dorsal fins that fit into the two slots cut into the resected talar surface. The UHMW polyethylene tibial component is also wider anteriorly. The two anterior holes in the prosthesis allow utilization of forceps or a hemostat to grasp the component to facilitate insertion or removal. The larger more lateral hole with a threaded surface accommodates the removable lever arm which facilitates handling, insertion, and removal. It is essential to position the units for proper alignment. The lever arm should project along an imaginary line between the first and second metatarsals or between the great and second toes. The serrated nonarticular surface of the tibial component has a single dorsal fin that fits into a rectangular osteotomy slot previously cut into the resected tibial surface. This oblique medial surface is designed to eliminate a sharp right angle osteotomy cut in the medial malleolar area which helps to protect against stress or fatigue fractures which could occur in this area with weight bearing forces. The pressures are then more evenly dissipated over the bone interface of the tibia. Two metallic wires are embedded in the structure of the UHMW prosthesis to help ascertain roentgenographic alignment. The ankle comes in a right and left model and "one size fits all adults."

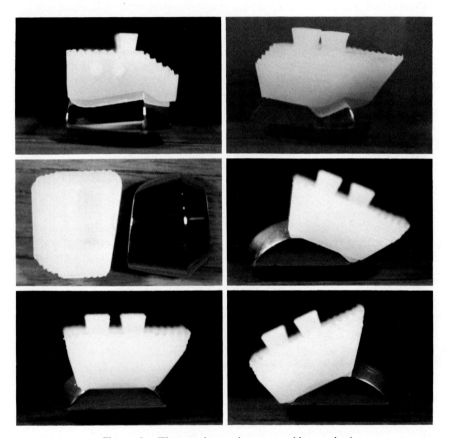

Figure 1. The angular total contact ankle prosthesis.

## INSTANT CENTERS OF ROTATION AND SURFACE VELOCITIES

The ankle (like the knee) has a multiple changing or instant center of rotation. The talus is considered the stationary member and the tibia the moving member. Sammarco et al.[15] have shown that the continually changing instant center of rotation that occurs from the time motion is begun in flexion to its termination in extension normally lies scattered in the body of the talus as well as anterior and inferior to the talus (Fig. 2). It was previously considered that the tibiotalar joint had only a single or even double axis of rotation but this is no longer valid. The lines representing surface velocity (direction) should be tangent to the contact point of the talar surface. Any abnormal axis of rotation or surface velocity other than those necessary for normal flexion and extension could well lead to excessive prosthetic wear and loosening. The normal ankle has a tendency toward distraction early in motion followed by a sliding throughout the midportion and ends in compression at the end of dorsiflexion. This compression could account for some of the tibial osteophytes noted on the neck of the talus seen on some of the roentgenograms in the case reports.

The process reverses itself when the joint moves in the opposite direction. In the prosthetic components the articular surfaces seem to be in a constant gliding contact and all relative motion seems to proceed smoothly during motion utilized in ambulation. These salient points have received the most important consideration in the design of the

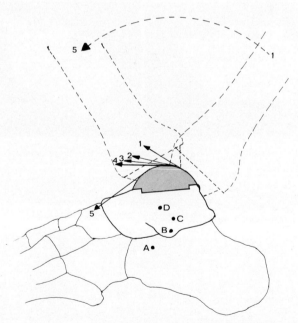

Figure 2.   Instant centers of motion (A to D) and surface velocities (1 to 5).

prosthetic models so that only a recapitulation of tibiotalar motion is simulated.

## NORMAL ANKLE MOTION, GAIT, AND PROSTHETIC COMPARISON

The tibiofibular-talar joint has been considered for many years as an example of a trochlear joint.[2, 8] This hinge-like or pulley motion depends upon the sliding of the tibia across the talus. What constitutes normal "ankle" motion has created a deluge of confusion in various reports over the years. Tibiopedal motion generally denotes the entire composite foot and ankle motion which includes not only the tibiofibular-talar or "true ankle joint" but also motion of all the tarsal bones as well. Tibiotalar motion then should imply only motion of flexion and extension between the tibial and talar articular surfaces. Because of this overlap of terms and the subsequent confusion it is probably wise to be more specific in terminology when referring to the "ankle joint." The range of motion for normal tibiotalar joints, both weight bearing and non-weight bearing, is then much less than reported by previous investigators. This may be perhaps explained in that external measurements register the composite tibiopedal articular motion and cannot isolate true tibiotalar motion. Studies on cadaver nonviable tissue and on ankle joints stripped of soft tissue[11] to study motion which has removed their restraining functions have also had a tendency to confuse this issue. Murry, Drought, and Kory[14] measured tibiopedal motion in adult men aged 20 to 65 walking in shoes. Their values were ascertained by placing silver tape markers on the shoe and then obtaining motion photographic studies of the subject correlating to the stance and swing phases of a walking cycle. Stance phase normally occupies 60 per cent of the walking cycle. The cycle that begins at heel-strike is followed by a short, sharp, flexion of approximately 10 degrees which permits contact of the entire foot with the floor. This foot-flat phase allows for a larger base of support providing for the weight of the oncoming body. The leg then rotates over the fixed foot and the ankle begins to extend. This slow and steady extension reaches its maximum during the midstance phase at approximately 40 per cent of the walking cycle but never exceeds 10 degrees. When the knee is beginning its major flexion movements the ankle reciprocally reverses from extension to flexion. Plantar flexion then becomes more rapid at 50 per cent of the cycle as the heel is elevated.

This flexion continues and reaches its maximun at 65 per cent of the walking cycle when the toe has left the floor. The maximal plantar flexion following the heel and toe-off phases was recorded as never being greater than 25 degrees. The ankle then promptly extends to allow foot clearance during the swing phase and finally flexes gently in anticipation of the next heel strike. Wright et al.[22] demonstrated that plantar flexion may be entirely accomplished at the ankle joint. During dorsiflexion in the stance phase, however, tibial motion cannot entirely be resolved about the ankle axis and, therefore, internal rotation of the tibia about the fixed foot must act through the subtalar axis to produce pronation which is dorsiflexion, abduction, and eversion of the foot relative to the leg. In general the tibia internally rotates during the first 15 per cent of the cycle and externally rotates during the remainder of the stance phase. The tibiotalar and subtalar joints are independent but seemingly act as a single mechanism during walking. The mediolateral axis of the ankle is usually not quite parallel to that of the knee because of the torsion between the upper and lower ends of the tibia. The torsion is typically an external one so that the ankle joint is not normally at a right angle to the line of progression. The ankle axis is externally rotated in a horizontal plane and hence is oblique to the frontal plane of the foot. Eversion of the foot rotates the tibia internally bringing the axis more nearly perpendicular to the plane of progression and inversion does the opposite. Rotation of the tibia produced by the inverted or everted foot positions affect the knee as well as the ankle joint just as alternations of the femur, knee, and tibia affect ankle rotation and foot position. These concepts may then be utilized when evaluating the results of a prosthetic replacement arthroplasty to the intricate function and motion of a normal tibiofibular-talar joint. A case report of the first total ankle replacement accomplished in this series and the results some two years later help demonstrate an analysis of the motion, stability, and function of the prosthetic joint in weight bearing maneuvers:

CASE 1. A 55 year old white male farmer was evaluated for a very painful right ankle on March 3, 1972. A vague history of trauma while driving a tractor was obtained. This probably represented a joint involved with osteoarthritis aggravated by trauma, as the opposite ankle also had a moderate amount of osteoarthritis. In December of 1971 an arthrotomy was performed. The procedure was unknown and the ankle remained painful. The patient resorted to crutches. In March, 1972 a second arthrotomy was done by the author to debride the joint, remove the hypertrophic osteophytic anterior tibia margin, in addition to the synovectomy. Tissue cultures were obtained and no infection could be demonstrated. The results of the second arthrotomy were poor (Fig. 3).

The patient continued to use crutches and walked with an antalgic gait. Physical therapy, local steroid injections, and oral nonsteroid antiphlogistic agents were utilized with only limited benefits. Because of the persistent painful symptoms and the difficulty of performing farm work while using crutches (for approximately two years) the arthritic tibiotalar joint was resected and replaced with a prosthetic total ankle. A gait analysis of the involved ankle and foot with corresponding roentgenograms is demonstrated (Fig. 4). The motion of the ankle during the stance phase of a walking cycle is depicted and corresponds very well to the patient's contralateral ankle (Fig. 5). A series of views (Fig. 6) also demonstrates the comparison of motion and stability of the prosthetic ankle to the left ankle in standing flat, on the toes and heels, as well as pronation and supination. The results have been very gratifying. The patient works full time on his farm without any restrictions, has no pain, and does not utilize crutches or cane.

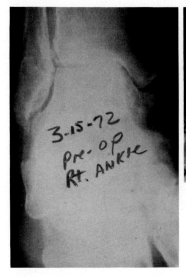
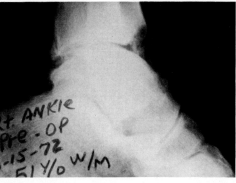

Figure 3. A 55 year old farmer in whom two previous arthrodeses failed to debride the right ankle joint. The ankle remained painful and the patient used crutches for over two years.

## CLINICAL MATERIAL

The present series included 31 ankles in 30 patients operated on for advanced arthritis of the ankle joint between April, 1973 and November, 1974. Replacement arthroplasties were performed on the right in 18 ankles, on the left in 13, and bilaterally in 1. The ages of the patients ranged from 17 to 70. Sixteen patients were male and 14 were female. Of the 30 patients, 20 (66.67 per cent) had traumatic degenerative arthritis, 6 (20 per cent) had rheumatoid arthritis and 4 (13.33 per cent) had primary osteoarthritis. As would be surmised a relatively younger group comprised the traumatic group with an average age of 41, as compared to those with rheumatoid arthritis with an average age of 62, and age 61 for the primary osteoarthritic group. The majority of the patients are being followed on an outpatient basis in the clinic. No patients are included in this series which had operations performed in other medical centers. No joints have been removed to arthrodese the joint nor has any primary deep surgical infection developed to date. One prosthesis (the early type model tibial component) became loose from an improper alignment which necessitated an additional procedure to correctly reposition the components.

## OPERATIVE TECHNIQUE

The usual preoperative and operative preparation is identical to that utilized for total hip and knee replacement arthroplasty procedures

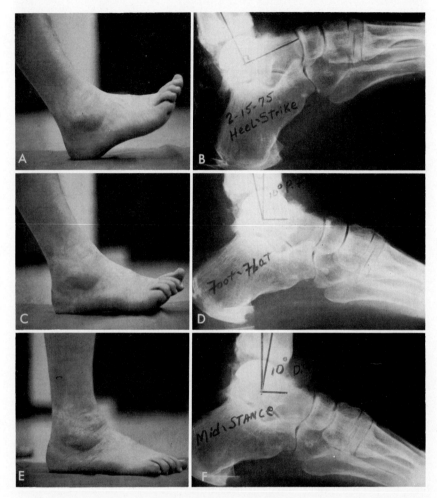

Figure 4.   A gait analysis of tibiopedal motion of the prosthetic ankle of this patient some two years later with duplicating roentgenograms in comparable positions projected in a simulated stance phase of gait. The stance phase occupies approximately 60 per cent of a walking cycle. *A* and *B*, Heel-strike initiates the stance phase. *C* and *D*, Foot-flat phase. Following heel-strike there is a short, sharp plantar flexion of the foot of approximately 10 degrees. *E* and *F*, Midstance phase. Following the foot-flat phase the leg rotates over the fixed foot and the ankle begins to extend. This slow and steady extension reaches its maximum during mid-stance or around 40 per cent of the walking cycle but never exceeds 10 degrees of dorsiflexion (extension).

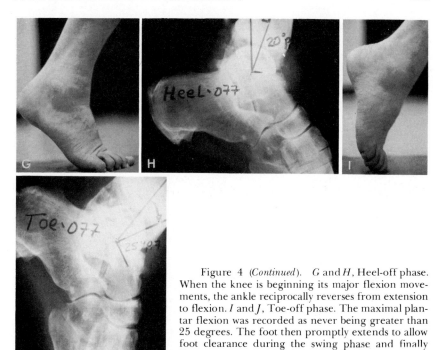

Figure 4 (*Continued*). *G* and *H*, Heel-off phase. When the knee is beginning its major flexion movements, the ankle reciprocally reverses from extension to flexion. *I* and *J*, Toe-off phase. The maximal plantar flexion was recorded as never being greater than 25 degrees. The foot then promptly extends to allow foot clearance during the swing phase and finally flexes again in anticipation of heel-strike.

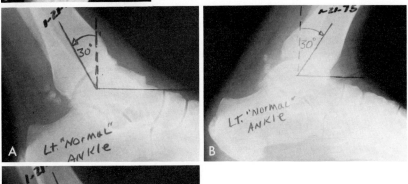

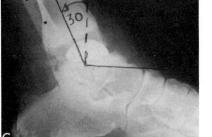

Figure 5. The motion of the prosthetic ankle (*C*) compares favorably with motion of the contralateral ankle (*A* and *B*). Maximal weight bearing, flexion and extension, is 30 degrees of the normal ankle, and the total ankle replacement recapitulates this motion.

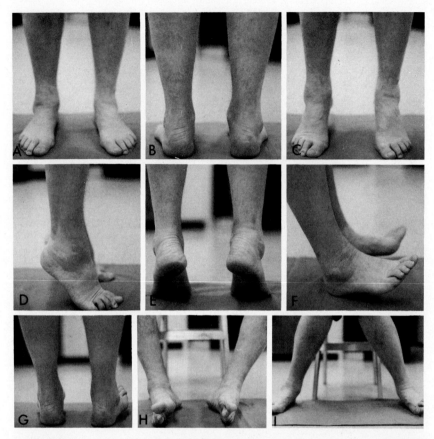

Figure 6.  *A* to *G*, Various weight bearing maneuvers demonstrated the projected intrinsic stability of the total ankle prosthetic units in the foot—flat-standing, toe-standing, and heel-standing position. *H* to *I*. Weight bearing stability in a varus and valgus attitude.

including laboratory studies. Weight bearing views of the foot and ankle are obtained for later comparison views in the postoperative phase. A marking pencil is used to outline the incision.

The operative procedures are outlined diagrammatically in Figure 7. A "lazy-S" curvilinear incision facilitates an anterior exposure. The incision starts on the anteromedial aspect of the ankle, curves gently in an oblique manner across the tibiotalar joint and then distally along the anterolateral aspect of the dorsum of the foot. (Alternate routes to expose the joint can be utilized if necessary such as the transfibular approach.) The interval between the anterior tibial and the extensor hallucis longus tendons is developed into the ankle joint. It is considered important to leave as much soft tissue covering deep to the extensor tendons as possible. This soft tissue is closed at the end of the procedure. This helps to cover the prosthetic components, decrease dead space, and perhaps minimize cicatrix formation which would tend to decrease motion.

The reciprocating power saw is used to remove a rectangular portion of the tibia perpendicular to the long axis of the tibia, as marked by the trial gauge ankle template. Then a similar portion of the dome of the talus is removed *parallel* to the tibial surface as outlined by the trial gauge block. Careful attention must be given to placement of the foot in a neutral position before resecting the talar dome. If the foot is in an equinus position a posterior capsulotomy can be done which allows bringing the foot into a neutral positon. An Achilles tendon lengthening should be deferred for obvious reasons to allow early postoperative motion. If the tibial or talar surfaces are not resected perpendicular to the sagittal plane of the tibia and talus with the foot in a neutral position difficulties in proper alignment could be encountered with contemplated loss of motion in either flexion or extension. A varus or valgus tilt might create an abnormal heel position. The trial gauge block is inserted to determine if the space is adequate and to check alignment. It should fit snugly into the prepared cavity and the lever arm should project between the first and second metatarsals. Slots in the template are marked to facilitate removing small rectangular osteotomy slots from the talus and tibia to accommodate the nonarticular stabilizing projections of the prosthetic components. One slot is necessary in the tibia and two in the talus. After the slots are made in the tibia and talus the trial prosthesis is inserted and the prosthetic components should articulate snugly. Operative roentgenograms are helpful at this time with the prosthetic components in place.

The foot can usually be distracted to facilitate easy insertion or removal of the components. The removable lever arm of the tibial component should project toward the first and second metatarsal area. Motion and position must be carefully checked.

Holes are also drilled or curetted into the tibia and talus to facilitate methacrylate purchase. The tibial component is initially seated. It is helpful once the tibial component is positioned and excessive soft cement trimmed to insert the talar component (without cement) which helps maintain the desired position and seat the tibial component with pressure while the foot is held in a neutral position. Often excessive posterior joint cement can be removed if sponges moistened in saline are packed in the posterior joint space prior to seating of the prosthesis and then carefully removed along the medial and lateral gutters while the methacrylate is in the doughy stage. The talar component is then removed, the tibial component checked for stability, and the process repeated while seating the talar component. Again, the removal of sponges carefully packed in the posterior joint and along the medial and lateral gutters prior to seating of the prosthesis help remove excessive cement. The ankle is then checked for stability and motion.

Operative x-ray films are necessary at this time. If clinical motion is impeded or if there is x-ray evidence of a posterior bolus of cement a posteromedial approach can be made for its removal. The ankle is then drained with a closed suction tube and closed carefully in layers. A closure of soft tissues deep to the tendons is desirable for previously stated reasons. A short leg cotton cast is applied with outer plaster of Paris to maintain the ankle in a neutral position.

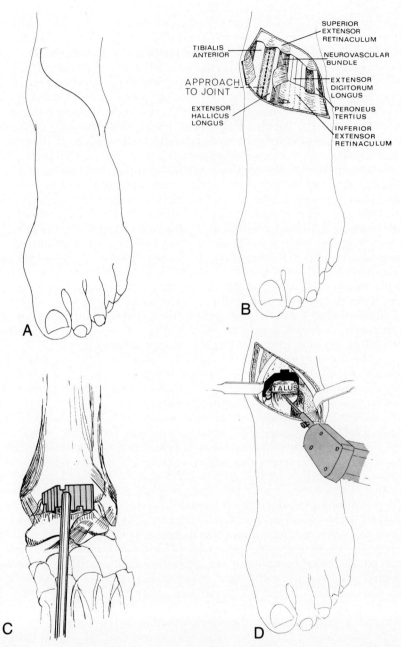

Figure 7. *A*, The ankle is exposed through an anterior "lazy-S" incision. *B*, The interval developed into the joint is between the anterior tibial and extensor hallucis longus tendons. *C*, A trial block gauge helps determine the amount of bone and configuration of the osteotomies. It should fit snugly into the resected surfaces and the long lever arm should project between the first and second metatarsals. This compensates for tibial torsion and helps project the articular components to the line of progression of the body. *D*, A reciprocating saw removes the desired portion and configuration of respective surfaces of the tibia and dome of talus.

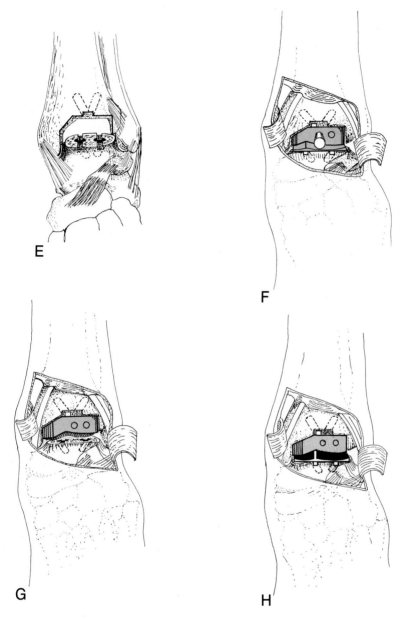

Figure 7 *(Continued)*.   *E*, The configuration of the resected tibial and talar surfaces. A single slot is cut into the tibia and two into the talus. Holes are projected into the surfaces for added purchase of methacrylate. The trial gauge block should fit snugly into this space. *F*. The trial components are inserted to check alignment and motion. The removable lever arm should project toward an interval between the great and second toes. *G*, The tibial component is cemented initially. The removable lever arm can also be utilized to position the prosthesis. The trial talar component may be slipped beneath the cemented tibial component to maintain pressure while the cement hardens with the foot in a neutral to slight dorsiflexed position and then removed. *H*, The talar component is then cemented into place.

## POSTOPERATIVE MANAGEMENT

The extremity is kept in an elevated postion and the suction tubing is removed in 24 to 48 hours. Isometric quadriceps sitting exercises and isotonic straight leg raising exercises are encouraged while in bed, as well as active knee motion. The cotton plaster cast is removed in five days and active motion and hydrotherapy begun in physical therapy. Protected partial weight bearing is encouraged until the discomfort subsides. Oral steroids are often helpful once range of motion activities are begun.

Full weight bearing is usually permitted by the time of dismissal unless the periarticular tissues remain painful after the newly acquired motion. If so, the patient should be dismissed on protected weight bearing until the symptoms subside. The patient with a preoperative equinus deformity due to contractures of the triceps surae musculature and posterior capsular tissues, especially noted in the traumatic group, have posed a special problem. These deformities cannot be stretched out preoperatively because of the joint incongruity. It has been possible, however, to get the ankles in these patients to at least a neutral position during surgery with a posterior capsulotomy, prior to insertion of the prosthesis. Heel cord lengthening has not been found to be necessary because once prosthetic joint congruity is established the heel cord can be effectively stretched. Motion has usually continued to improve after hospital dismissal with continued passive stretching and ambulation.

## ASSESSMENT OF RESULTS

From the standpoint of objective evaluation of results a weighted point system for grading has been developed. This has allowed an integrated, objective evaluation, taking into account all of the important functional considerations. This point system is outlined in Table 1.

## GRADING OF RESULTS

The major emphasis of this point system has been centered on pain evaluation and functional activities. A result was considered excellent if the point range was from 23 to 36, good from 16 to 22, fair from 11 to 15, and poor from 10 or below. In the present series the results were approximately 20 per cent excellent, 60 per cent good, 13.4 per cent fair, and 6.6 per cent poor in patients to date. The majority of patients are fully ambulatory without aid of crutch or cane and have a heel-toe stance phase gait pattern. Range of motion, as measured in postoperative weight bearing roentgenograms, has been sufficient to allow normal gait patterns and some approximate the same motion as the opposite uninvolved ankle. Motion seems to improve with the passage of time and with

**Table 1.**  *Evaluation of Results by Point System*

| | Point |
|---|---|
| *Pain* | |
| None | 12 |
| Slight, occasional, no compromise in activity | 8 |
| Mild, no effect on ordinary activity, pain after unusual activity | 6 |
| Moderate, tolerable, makes concessions, not improved | 3 |
| Marked, serious limitations, worse than before surgery | 0 |
| *Postoperative Motion* | |
| Normal to major improvement—70 per cent of motion as compared with contralateral ankle | 8 |
| Moderate improvement—50 per cent of motion as compared with contralateral ankle | 5 |
| Limited improvement—30 per cent of motion as compared with contralateral ankle | 3 |
| No improvement—10 per cent of motion as compared with contralateral ankle | 0 |
| *Functional Activities* | |
| Normal as desired, no limp or support | 8 |
| Some limitation, limp only with fatigue, does not use crutch or cane | 5 |
| Moderate limitation of desired activities such as walking up or down stairs and uneven surfaces, limp, uses cane or crutches occasionally | 3 |
| Serious limitations of function, limp, has to resort to crutches or cane, needs external support | 0 |
| *Work or Usual Occupation* | |
| Full time without difficulty | 8 |
| Full time with difficulty | 5 |
| Part time without difficulty | 3 |
| Part time with difficulty | 2 |
| Unable because of pain or limited motion | 0 |

Based on this point system a tabulation of results is made according to categories.

| | |
|---|---|
| Excellent | 23 - 36 |
| Good | 16 - 22 |
| Fair | 11 - 15 |
| Poor | 10 or less |

continued usage, as would be suspected. The procedure has generally eliminated pain in the ankle joint.

A few patients have discomfort, localized either in the medial or lateral ligamentous area or in the posterior heel area, which has a tendency to subside with time. No ankle appears unstable during weight bearing stress nor is any instability noted in walking up or down or laterally on inclined surfaces. There have been no infections but two patients have had superficial marginal wound necrosis that healed with local wound care. No ankles have had to be arthrodesed. Most patients have been able to return to their desired occupations such as farming, manual labor, teaching, waiting tables, etc. They are able to walk on uneven ground, up and down stairs, carry weighted objects, dance, and carry out other desired activities.

Of the two patients classified as having a poor result one had concomitant subtalar traumatic degenerative arthritic changes with a posteromedial talar nonunion fragment in additon to improper varus seating of the prosthetic unit. This resulted in a varus heel position, however the ankle motion was good. This abnormal heel and prosthetic position eventually resulted in the talar component becoming loose. The problem has been corrected by a repositioning of the prosthesis and a fibular osteotomy which, in retrospect, should have been done prior to the replacement arthroplasty. The second patient obtained a poor result because of excessive scar tissue about the ankle joint which could not be corrected at the time of surgery or with secondary soft tissue releases. This patient does not complain of pain, however, and motion might improve with time and usage.

## COMPLICATIONS

There have been no major complications to date. One patient revealed a delayed staphylococcus coagulase-positive growth on tissue cultures, made from tissue removed from the joint at the time of surgery (despite a negative gram stain report received in surgery). No postoperative infection has developed in over 18 months in this patient. Two patients have had superficial marginal wound necrosis. No systemic complications have been recognized. Careful laboratory studies including enzyme and liver profile evaluations preoperatively and postoperatively are routinely obtained and no abnormalities have been detected. The various complications noted in other joints such as the hip and knee replaced with similar components are appreciated and could well manifest a problem in the ankle in the future.

## CLINICAL EXPERIENCE

CASE 1. A 55 year old white male geologist sustained a comminuted fracture of his right ankle approximately 25 years ago. Previous surgical procedures were unsuccessful and a painful, traumatic, arthritic joint with a varus instability resulted. The patient had refused previous recommendations to have the ankle arthrodesed. An osteotomy of the fibula with internal osteosynthesis and screw fixation helped stabilize the joint but painful, limited motion remained (Fig. 8). A total ankle replacement arthroplasty was subsequently performed that resulted in a functional stable ankle joint with excellent painless motion. The patient is now able to work and engage in desired sports and other functional activities without difficulty in the involved ankle.

CASE 2.    A 38 year old white female nurse sustained injuries to her right ankle joint that resulted in traumatic arthritis. The ankle was painful and had limited motion (Fig. 9). The patient walked on her toes in an equinus attitude. A total ankle replacement arthroplasty was performed in addition to a posterior capsulotomy. Triceps surae tenotomy, and lengthening, was unnecessary. The patient now works full time and engages in desired activities without pain and had a normal heel-toe plantargrade stance phase of tibiopedal motion.

CASE 3.    A 51 year old white female secretary had a painful traumatic left ankle for several years which was unresponsive to all conservative management. The patient utilized crutches and walked with an equinus attitude of the foot and ankle. A total ankle replacement was done which resulted in a functional ankle joint with comparable motion to the contralateral ankle (Fig. 10). The patient ambulates without the aid of crutches or cane and has no pain or restrictions in the involved ankle.

CASE 4.    A 65 year old self-employed white male fell from the roof of his home and sustained a comminuted fracture of the right ankle in addition to depressed tibial plateau fractures. Open reduction and internal osteosynthesis of the ankle fractures failed (Fig. 11). No infection was present. The screw and broken Steinmann pins were removed and the arthritic joint resected and replaced by a prosthetic ankle joint. Gram stains obtained in surgery revealed no bacteria. However, late culture reports revealed a delayed staphylococcus coagulase-positive growth on tissue cultures despite the negative gram stain at surgery.

No infection is in evidence 18 months postoperatively, however. The ankle remained painful at the time of hospital dismissal so the patient utilized crutches for four months. Motion has gradually improved and pain has now subsided completely. The patient's only complaint presently is discomfort in the opposite ankle which is involved with minimal osteoarthritis and a dorsal compression osteophyte. The motion in the prosthetic ankle is slightly more than the opposite ankle. The patient had no restrictions in desired activities and walks without the aid of a crutch or cane.

CASE 5.    A 21 year old white male postgraduate student fell from a water tower and sustained a comminuted fracture of the foot and ankle with a loss of talar bone substance. No infection was present. The patient refused ankle arthrodesis recommendations. An initial subtalar arthrodesis was done to stabilize the remaining bone substance. Subsequently the destroyed joint was replaced with a prosthetic ankle (Fig. 12). The patient is now fully ambulatory without pain and motion is slowly improving. The midtarsal articulation appears stable with weight bearing.

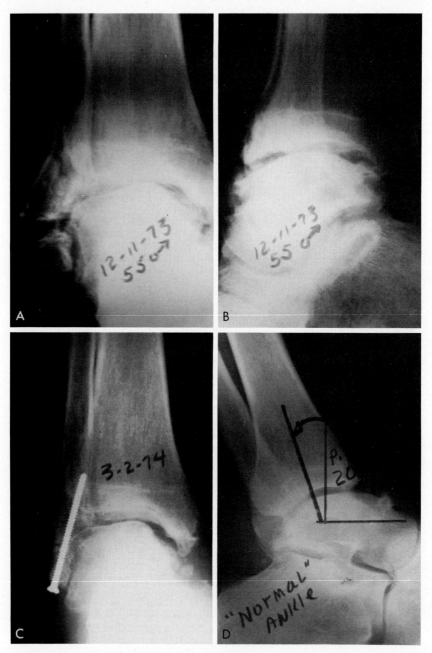

Figure 8. *A* and *B*, Comminuted fracture of right ankle sustained 25 years previously. Previous surgical procedures were unsuccessful and resulted in a painful, unstable, traumatic arthritic joint. *C*, Osteotomy of the fibula with screw internal osteosynthesis helped stabilize the joint but painful limited motion remained. *D* to *G*, Total ankle replacement arthroplasty resulted in excellent stable motion and pain has been eliminated. Plantar flexion in weight bearing projections is 25 degrees as compared with only 20 degrees in the opposite ankle which reveals a compression osteophyte on the anterior margin of the talus. *H*, Dorsiflexion is equal in both ankles and the frontal view in weight bearing reveals a stable prosthetic joint.

124

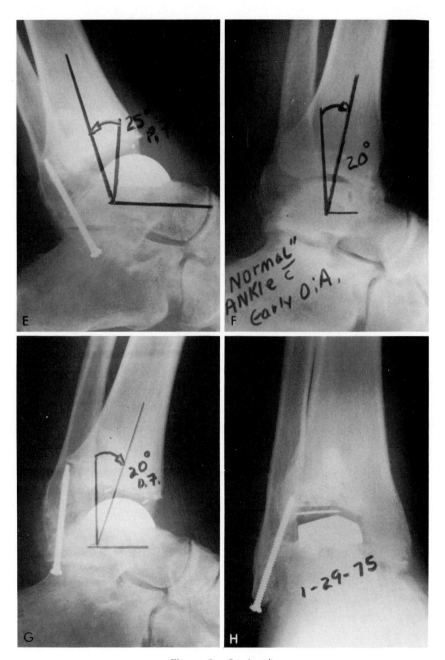

Figure 8 (*Continued*).

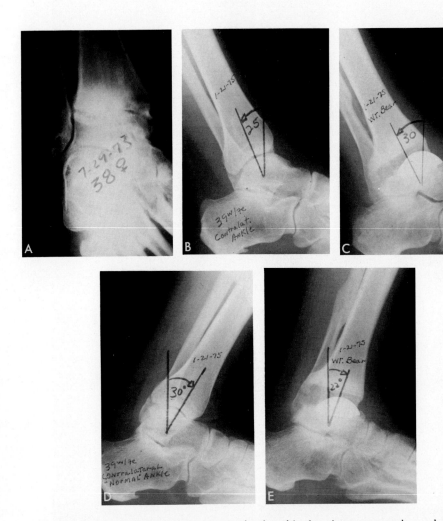

Figure 9. *A*, Posterior contractures developed in the triceps surae and capsular tissues so that the patient walked on her toes in an equinus position. *B* to *E*, A posterior capsulotomy was done at the time of replacement arthroplasty. The contracted triceps surae has been effectively corrected by passive stretching and heel-toe plantigrade ambulation. Plantar flexion is now to 30 degrees as compared to 25 degrees in the contralateral ankle and 22 degrees of plantar flexion as compared to 30 degrees in the normal ankle.

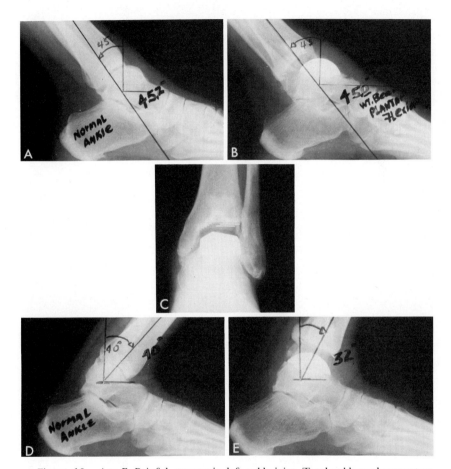

Figure 10. *A* to *E*, Painful, traumatic, left ankle joint. Total ankle replacement resulted in a functional, stable joint with comparable motion to the contralateral ankle.

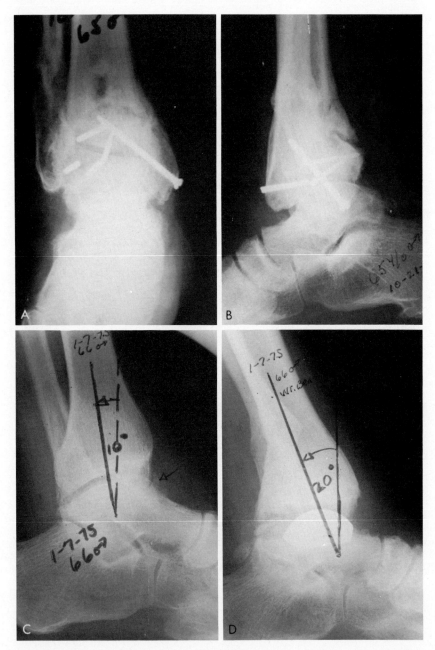

Figure 11.   *A* and *B*, Comminuted ankle fracture. *C* to *F*, Motion has gradually improved. (Note the original model prosthesis.)

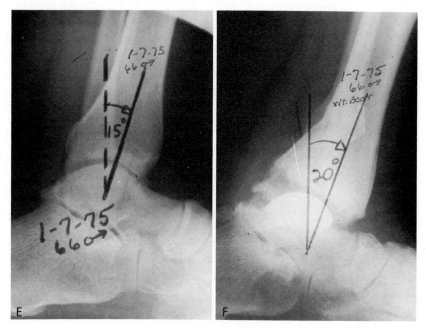

Figure 11 (*Continued*).

CASE 6. A 53 year old minister had a very painful right ankle of five years' duration with no history of antecedent trauma. A large cystic lesion is present in the talus in addition to smaller cystic areas along the articular surfaces (Fig. 13) in this apparent osteoarthritic joint. The patient was previously extremely obese and had a previous small bowel conduit circuit procedure with successful weight reduction of approximately 125 pounds. Admission routine chest roentgenograms and laboratory studies were normal. A total ankle arthroplasty was done to replace the arthritic joint. The cyst was curetted and filled with methacrylate. Operative gram stains of the joint fluid revealed no organisms. Delayed culture reports have revealed the presence of coccidioidomycosis. Internal medicine and rheumatology consultants have failed to detect the systemic source of this apparent disseminated pathogen. A decision has been made not to administer amphotericin B therapy. The patient is now back to full time ministry and walks without the aid of crutch or cane. Motion is slowly improving and discomfort is subsiding. There has been no evidence of any joint infection. Some consideration will be given to isolation of the extremity and extracorpal perfusion with appropriate medications if such a problem arises in the future.

CASE 7. A 61 year old white female school teacher had advanced rheumatoid arthritis changes of the left ankle and right knee. A prosthetic knee replacement arthroplasty was initially performed followed later with an ankle replacement arthroplasty. The results have been satisfactory to eliminate pain and restore function so that the patient has now returned to full time teaching. The tibial component was positioned with an anterior tilt of 15 degrees so that some motion was mechanically lost in plantar flexion (Fig. 14). This has not caused a problem clinically however.

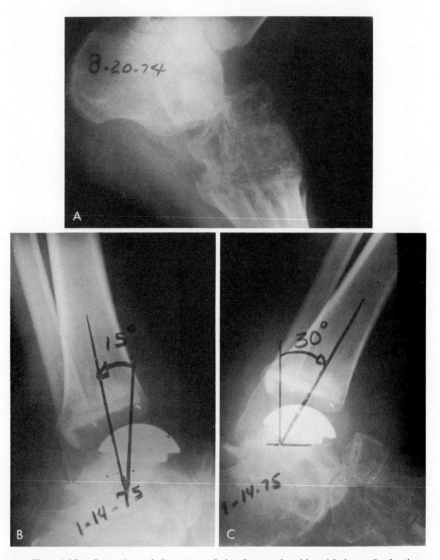

Figure 12. Comminuted fractures of the foot and ankle with loss of talar bone substance. *A*, Subtalar arthrodesis was done initially to protect the remaining bone. *B* and *C*, Later the destroyed joint was replaced with a prosthetic ankle.

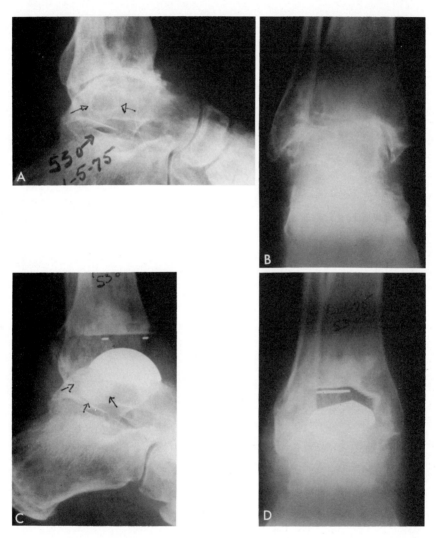

Figure 13. *A* and *B*, Painful right ankle for over five years with no antecedent history of trauma. A large "cystic" lesion is noted on the talus between the two arrows. *C* and *D*, The arthritic joint was resected and replaced with a prosthetic joint. The cyst was curetted and packed with methacrylate.

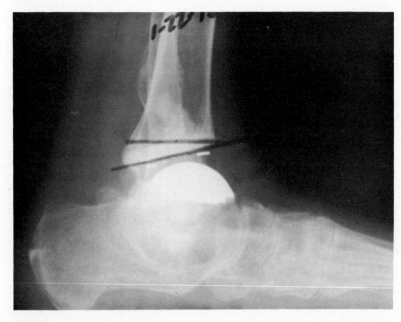

Figure 14.   The tibial component was positioned with an excessive (15 degree) anterior tilt so mechanically some motion was lost in plantar flexion.

CASE 8.   A 17 year old female sustained a comminuted left ankle fracture three years previously that resulted in a painful joint with limited motion. She had refused several recommendations to have the ankle stabilized and preferred crutches instead. The patient was referred by another orthopedist for replacement arthroplasty. Results have been poor despite good initial postoperative motion. A portion of the posteromedial talus was removed at the time of the arthroplasty for management of an avascular fragment and nonunion (Fig. 15). The heel was in a varus position clinically despite the contralateral ankle which also appears to be in a similar position. The talar component was seated with excessive anterior tilt which mechanically impeded a degree of dorsiflexion. Clinical motion was not impeded however. The patient over the next year worked as a waitress. Eventually the patient developed pain and a "click" in the joint. This problem might have been accentuated when the patient injured her ankle while practicing ballet. The talar component had loosened. The problem has now been corrected with a fibular osteotomy and repositioning of the components. The patient has resumed her full activities and no further difficulties have been encountered.

## DISCUSSION

There seems to be a rather large group of patients with advanced arthritic changes of the ankle joints who desire to have restoration of motion rather than a stabilizing arthrodesis as shown by the number of cases, 30 in approximately two years. As surmised, a relatively younger patient fell into the traumatic group. Relative ages for the osteoarthritic and the rheumatoid patients were similar to candidates for hip and knee replacement arthroplasties.

Thirty patients who were considered candidates for arthrodesis were selected for total ankle replacement arthroplasties. One patient had bilateral procedures after initial subtalar arthrodesis. In general, the pain has been totally eliminated or modified so that it has not posed a problem after the immediate postoperative period. Function has been vastly improved and stability has not been a problem due to prosthetic design and ligamentous support of the ankle which has been left intact. Motion of the joint has generally been enough to allow a normal heel-toe gait pattern and to allow ambulation without a limp. Superimposed

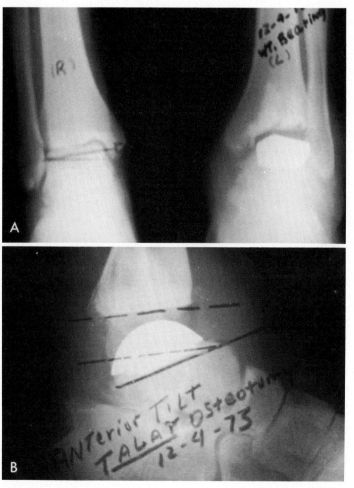

Figure 15. *A* and *B*, Comminuted left ankle fracture. A nonviable posteromedial bone fragment was removed from the talus at the time of replacement arthroplasty.

roentgenograms of weight bearing ankle motion studies revealed an active range of motion of 30 to 40 degrees in flexion and extension which in many cases compared favorably with that noted in the opposite ankle. Motion of the ankle joint also depends on the degree of surrounding soft tissue scarring, muscle contractures, and so forth, and as expected should improve with proper exercise and usage once the soft tissues have reached a state of equilibrium. Arthrodesis can still be carried out as a salvage medium should it be indicated in the future. No prostheses have had to be removed for ankle arthrodesis, however. Weight bearing loads have had no demonstrable effect on the bone interface surfaces. The many problems noted to occur in the hip and knee replacement arthroplasties are appreciated and, of course, may occur in the ankle joint at a later date. The ankle joint appears to be a suitable recipient for total replacement prosthetic procedures and is similar to the hip joint in this respect.

## CONCLUSION

Total ankle replacement is not a panacea for all ankle problems. On the basis of a relatively small series followed for a relative short period of time, however, we have been impressed with the possibilities and believe that total joint replacement should be considered when planning any surgical treatment for advanced arthritic changes which have resulted in pain, loss of motion, and disability of the ankle joint.

## REFERENCES

1. Amstuz, H. C.: Biomaterials for artificial joints. Orthop. Clin. North Amer., 4:235-248, 1973.

2. Barnett, C. H., Davis, D. V., and Macconaill, M.D.: Synovial joints: their structure and mechanics. Springfield, Charles C Thomas, 1961, pp. 163-169.

3. Cahoon, J. R., and Paxton, H. W.: A metallurgical survey of current orthopedic implants. J. Biomed. Mater. Res., 4:223-244, 1970.

4. Charnley. J.: Acrylic Cement in Orthopedic Surgery. Baltimore, Williams and Wilkins Co., 1970.

5. Charnley, J.: The long term results of low-friction arthroplasty of the hip performed as a primary intervention. J. Bone Joint Surg., 56B:61-76, 1972.

6. Charosky, C. B., Bullough, P. G., and Wilson, P. D., Jr.: Total hip replacement failures: A histological evaluation. J. Bone Joint Surg., 55A:49-58, 1973.

7. Close, J. R.: Some applications of the functional anatomy of the ankle joint. J. Bone Joint Surg., 38A:761-781, 1956.

8. Grant, J. C.: Boileau: A Method of Anatomy. Baltimore, Williams and Wilkins Co., 1958, pp.17-18.

9. Hague, M. F.: Knee in patients with hip joint ankylosis. Acta Orthop. Scand., 44:485-495, 1973.

10. Inman, V. T.: Influence on the ankle of the proximal limb. Artif. Limbs, 13:59-65, 1969.

11. Isman, R. E., and Inman, V. T.: Anthropometric studies of the human foot and ankle. Bull. Pros. Res., 10-11:97-129, 1969.

12. Kattles, J. F., and Field, M.: Surface integrity—A new requirement for surfaces generated by material—Removed methods. Proc. Inst. Mech. Engrs., 182:31-45, 1967-1968.

13. Laing, P. G.: Compatibility of biomaterials. Orthop. Clin. North Amer., 4:249-273, 1973.

14. Murry, M. P., Drought, A. B., and Kory, R. C.: Walking patterns in normal men. J. Bone Joint Surg., 46A:235-360, 1964.

15. Sammarco, G. J., Burstein, A. H., and Frankel, V.H.: Biomechanics of the ankle: A kinematic study. Orthop. Clin. North Amer., 4:75-96, 1973.

16. Scales, J. T., and Lowe, S. A.: Some Factors Influencing Bone and Joint Replacement. Philadelphia, J. B. Lippincott, 1971.

17. Scott, D.: Surface studies in the investigation of failure mechanisms. Proc. Inst. Mech. Engrs., 182:56-64, 1967.

18. Walker, P. S., and Erkman, M. J.: Metal-on-metal lubrication in artificial human joint wear. 21:377-392, 1972.

19. Walker, P. S., Salvati, E. A., and Hotzler, R. K.: The wear on removed McKee-Farrar total hip prostheses. J. Bone Joint Surg. 56A:92-100, 1974.

20. Walker, P. S., and Bullough, P. G.: The effects of friction and wear in artificial joints. Orthop. Clin. North Amer., 4:275-293, 1973.

21. Weseley, M. S., Koval, R., and Kleiger, B.: Roentgen measurement of ankle flexion-extension measurement. Clin. Orthop., 65:167-174, 1969.

22. Wright, D. G., Desai, S. M., and Henderson, W.: Action of the subtalar and ankle complex during the stance phase of walking. J. Bone Joint Surg., 46A:361-382, 1964.

*Chapter 9*

# Ankle Arthrodesis

HARRY D. MORRIS, M.D.*

RICHARD T. HERRICK, M.D.†

Ankle arthrodesis has been advocated since 1878[17, 37] to correct paralytic deformities. It is most frequently necessary in recent times to improve function after poor results of treatment of ankle fractures.[17, 31] At least 22 distinctly different techniques for arthrodesis have been described in the literature,[54] including nine specific approaches, each with several modifications suggested by various other authors, with apparently good results. This large number of procedures implies that no particular method has been quite satisfactory for most surgeons (Table 1).

Obviously not all surgeons have been able to duplicate the originator's results and each method has different complications or undesirable results. Important factors that affect the results are different indications, age, and general condition of the patient, whether internal fixation, or grafts, or both were used, and length and type of immobilization used.

A few authors have attempted to compare and contrast the results of the various procedures,[8, 9, 16, 17, 27, 31, 44, 47, 49, 52] but none has satisfactorily correlated the long-term results with indications, age, and sex of the patients, length and type of immobilization, previous operations, complications, and interval between onset of injury or disease, which this chapter attempts to do.

## MATERIAL AND METHODS

The records of all ankle fusions done at the Ochsner Medical Center from 1942 to 1973 were reviewed. A total of 63 ankle fusions were done on 54 patients (three patients had bilateral procedures). Five were repeat arthrodeses, the original having failed to produce a solid fusion, and another was done for a postoperative calcaneovalgus foot deformity. All

* Clinical Professor of Surgery (Orthopedics), Tulane University School of Medicine, New Orleans, Louisiana.
† Fellow in Orthopedic Surgery, Alton Ochsner Medical Foundation and Ochsner Clinic, New Orleans, Louisiana.

**Table 1.**   *The Major Approaches to Ankle Fusion and Percentage of*
*Solidly Fused Ankles as Found in the Literature*

| APPROACH | PERCENTAGE | REFERENCES |
|---|---|---|
| Transfibular | 90 | 1, 7, 9, 16, 19, 21, 25, 29, 31, 32, 40, 44, 49, 50, 51 |
| Medial | 100 | 41, 53 |
| Bilateral incisions | 92 | 5, 18, 29 |
| Transmalleolar | 96 | 2, 26, 27, 35 |
| Simple decortication | 100 | 8, 54 |
| Compression arthrodesis | 92 | 3, 8, 12, 17, 23, 27, 29, 34, 42, 48, 49 |
| Posterior | 94 | 16, 17, 31, 44, 47, 54 |
| Anterior | 91 | 7, 9, 10, 14, 16, 22, 24, 27-31, 33, 36-39, 44-47, 49, 52, 54 |
| Combined anterior and posterior | 100 | 11 |

patients who could be located were asked to answer a short questionnaire concerning results. Approximately 50 per cent responded to the questionnaires and 20 per cent were re-examined by one of the authors.

### Age and Sex Distribution

The ages of the patients at the time of operation ranged from eight to 67 years, with an average of 36.5 years and a median age of 37 years.

There were 29 primary procedures carried out on men and five of the repeat fusions and 28 primary procedures on women and one repeat. Thirty of the primary fusions and three repeat procedures were on the right; 27 primary fusions and three repeat procedures were done on the left.

### Interval and Length of Follow-up

The interval between the onset of symptoms and the initial fusion procedure ranged from two months to 48 years with an average of 7 years and a median of 3 years. Total length of follow-up of the patients ranged from three months to 24 years, with an average of 5.2 years and a median of 3.75 years. All patients were evaluated at regular intervals, if possible, until radiographic evidence of fusion was present.

### Indications

The most frequent (60 per cent) indication for arthrodesis of the ankle was for post-traumatic malfunctioning ankles. Earlier studies had a greater proportion of fusions done for post polio paralysis and tuberculosis, but only some of the earlier cases in this study were done for the former and none for the latter (Table 2). The presenting complaint was almost invariably a painful stiff ankle regardless of the causative factor.

**Table 2.**  *Indications for Arthrodesis*

| | | |
|---|---|---|
| Postfracture osteoarthritis | | 17 |
| Postfracture malunion or nonunion | | 13 |
| Osteoarthritis | | 2 |
| Rheumatoid arthritis | | 5 |
| Pseudarthrosis | | 6 |
| Paralytic feet | | 15 |
|     Post polio paralysis | 9 | |
|     Meningomyelocele | 4 | |
|     Paresis after herniated | | |
|       nucleus pulposis | 2 | |
| Clubfoot | | 2 |
| Cerebral palsy | | 1 |
| Charcot-Marie-Tooth disease | | 1 |
| Osteomyelitis | | 1 |

## Previous Operative Procedures

The most common previous operation was closed reduction of fractures, with open reduction and internal fixation of fractures and triple arthrodeses of the subtalar joint next in frequency (Table 3).

## Length and Type of Immobilization

The total length of immobilization ranged from one month to 10 months with an average of 4.7 months and a median of 4.25 months. The length of non-weight bearing immobilization ranged from zero months to eight months with an average of 2.1 months and a median of 1.75 months, both of which compare favorably with most previous studies. When any doubt of clinical fusion existed, the ankle was immobilized until there was radiographic evidence of bony bridging of the tibiotalar joint. The length of time between the definitive operation for arthrodesis and radiographic evidence of solid fusion ranged from two to 15 months, with an average of 5.2 months and a median of 4.0 months.

Various types of immobilization were used. Most commonly a short leg or long leg non-weight bearing plaster of Paris cast was applied for approximately one month, followed by a short leg non-weight bearing plaster of Paris cast for one month, and a short leg walking plaster of Paris cast for two months. In several instances immobilization was continued if there was any question of solid fusion with a short leg walking plaster of Paris cast or a short leg splint for an additional month or until at least clinical evidence of solid fusion existed.

## PROCEDURES AND RESULTS

The final results of ankle fusion procedures are very difficult to determine on a purely objective basis (Table 4). The ultimate goal for such

**Table 3.**  *Previous Operative Procedures*

| PROCEDURE | NUMBER |
|---|---|
| Closed reduction of fractures | 16 |
| Open reduction and internal fixation of fractures | 11 |
| Triple arthrodesis of foot | 12 |
| Attempted ankle arthrodesis | 6 |
| Tendo Achillis lengthening | 1 |
| Lumbrinudi procedure | 2 |
| Tendon transfers of the foot | 2 |

**Table 4.**  *Procedures and Results*

| PROCEDURE | NUMBER | RESULTS | | |
|---|---|---|---|---|
| | | Good | Fair | Poor |
| Sliding tibial graft and screws, etc. | 29 | 19 | 5 | 5 |
| Sliding tibial graft with Charnley compression device | 6 | 5 | 1 | 0 |
| Modified Charnley procedure | 8 | 6 | 0 | 2 |
| Anderson procedure | 5 | 1 | 3 | 1 |
| Anderson procedure with fibular graft | 2 | 1 | 0 | 1 |
| Simple tibiotalar coaption | 3 | 2 | 0 | 1 |
| Pantalar arthrodesis | 5 | 3 | 1 | 1 |
| Pantalar arthrodesis with Charnley compression device | 2 | 1 | 1 | 0 |
| Adams procedure | 3 | 3 | 0 | 0 |
| TOTAL | 63 | 41 | 11 | 11 |
| PER CENT | 100 | 65 | 17.5 | 17.5 |

procedures is to obtain a painless fusion in a functional limb, allowing the patient to perform the same activities as before the accident or onset of the disease. We classified the results as good, fair, or poor according to the following criteria: *Good*: A painless, clinically-solid ankle fusion with radiographic evidence of bony fusion, allowing the patient to perform usual daily activities without a limp. *Fair*: A solidly fused ankle clinically and radiographically that usually allowed performance of all activities but that occasionally exhibited limp and/or mild pain or swelling with extended prolonged stress. Also included in this category were all patients who required at least one more surgical procedure. *Poor*: All those not in the good or fair categories.

On this basis, the final results were 65 per cent good, 17.5 per cent fair (therefore 82.5 per cent satisfactory results) and 17 per cent poor results.

A possible improvement in these statistics could be produced if, as Baker[4] has suggested, the eight patients who exhibited a limp because of diminished tarsal motion were fitted with a solid ankle, cushion heel (SACH) and a metatarsal rocker on a steel-shanked shoe. This reportedly can improve the gait in otherwise successful ankle arthrodesis patients, and if so, would raise the percentage of good results from 65 per cent to 78 per cent (Fig. 1).

All fusions were attempted at no more than 5 degrees of equinus, preferably at the neutral position. All of the good results were within 5 degrees of the neutral position of flexion, never fixed in dorsiflexion, and all were in neutral version and rotation (Fig. 2).

Two of the female patients volunteered that they considered their ankles, although functionally satisfactory, to be esthetically unacceptable. This problem has only rarely been considered in the literature.[2, 26, 37, 39, 54] The bulbous shape of the fused ankle would perhaps be diminished by osteotomizing the malleoli, and this is reportedly[2, 27] of no detriment to the final result of ankle fusions. We have not used this method.

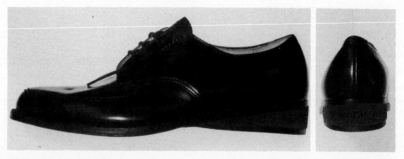

Figure 1. Solid ankle, cushion heel modified for a regular shoe which we have used on six patients, with improvement in gait and increased comfort, following arthrodesis of the ankle.

## Complications

The most common major complication was pseudarthrosis (6 patients or 9 per cent of the total patients). One death occurred after a transfusion reaction, which occurred very early in the series. One patient who underwent an arthrodesis for a pseudarthrosis from a previously attempted fusion was emotionally unstable, removed her own cast prematurely after the initial and second procedures, and eventually developed chronic osteitis and Charcot foot. There were three cases of chronic intractable osteomyelitis. One of these ultimately resulted in a below-knee amputation; the second was originally done in hope of eradicating an already infected ankle. The chronic iatrogenic infection rate was, therefore, 3 per cent, an acceptable figure in view of the fact that several of these patients underwent surgery in the very early antibiotic era.

There was a 26 per cent rate of major complications in the original 57 fusions, a 24 per cent rate of major complications considering all 63 procedures.

## DISCUSSION

There was no statistically significant relationship between the final result and the length and/or type of immobilization, however there was a definite tendency toward better results if non-weight bearing was adhered to for at least three months. In addition there was no statistically significant relationship between poor results and the method of arthrodesis used, although 82 per cent of the sliding anterior tibial grafts with any type of internal fixation had acceptable (good and fair) results (Fig. 3).

Age and sex of the patient did not seem to affect the final result, nor did the interval between onset of disease or initiating incident and the time of operation. The final result was almost always apparent six months postoperatively, and the ultimate result never changed from the status of the ankle 15 months after surgery.

## SUMMARY

Sixty-three cases of ankle arthrodesis using nine major surgical methods are presented. There were 82.5 per cent satisfactory results and 17.5 per cent poor. The most common complication was pseudarthroses (six patients). Age and sex of patient or interval between onset of disease or initiating incident and operation did not seem to affect the outcome.

The sliding anterior tibial graft with internal fixation is the method of choice (Fig. 4). It has been shown to produce pain-free, functional, fused ankles when correctly done for suitable indications and when non-weight bearing for six weeks or more and total immobilization for at least three months is employed.

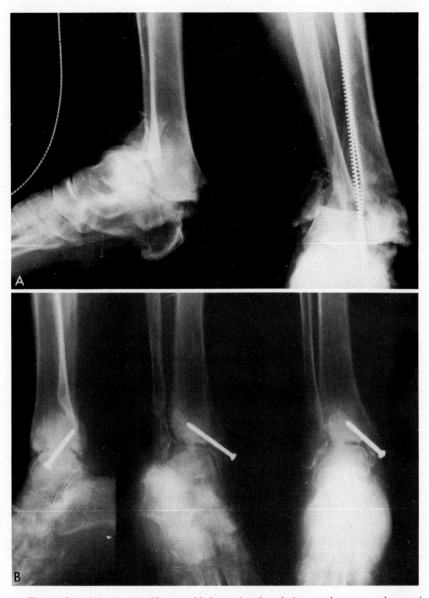

Figure 2. (Case 1) *A*, A 62 year old Caucasian female incurred compound comminuted fracture-dislocation, right ankle. This is the initial radiograph that was taken. *B*,
Radiograph taken four months post-injury. Debridement, open reduction, and internal
fixation of medial malleolus were carried out.

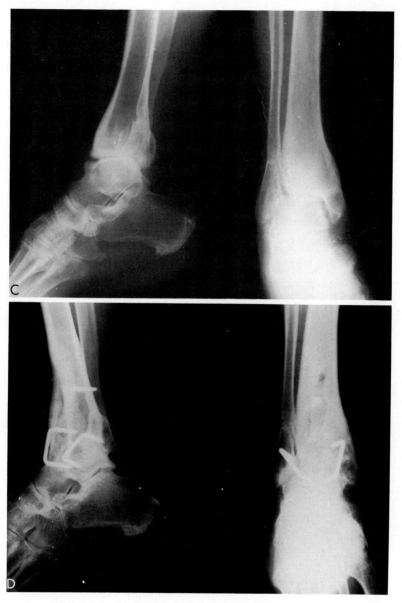

Figure 2 (*Continued*). *C*, Radiograph taken 40 months post-injury. Traumatic arthritis, loss of joint space, and equinus of foot were accompanied by severe pain. *D*, This radiograph was taken 15 months following arthrodesis of ankle. The patient is pain-free, has excellent gait, and can engage in full activity unsupported. The results of the arthrodesis were classified as good.

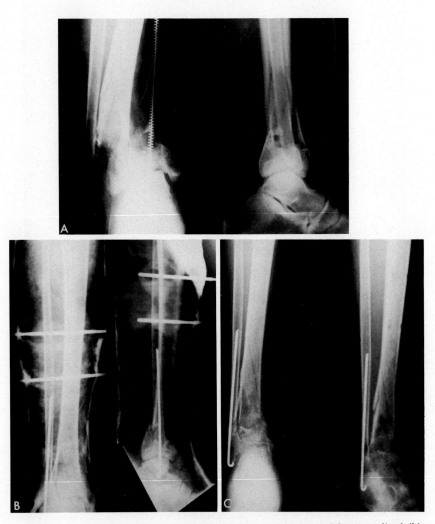

Figure 3. (Case 2) *A*, This is the initial x-ray film of a compound fracture, distal tibia and fibula, in a Caucasian male 40 years of age. *B*, This radiograph was taken three days post-injury following debridement, reduction, and internal fixation of fibula with Rush pin. *C*, A radiograph taken five months post-injury indicates presence of infection and delayed union of fractures.

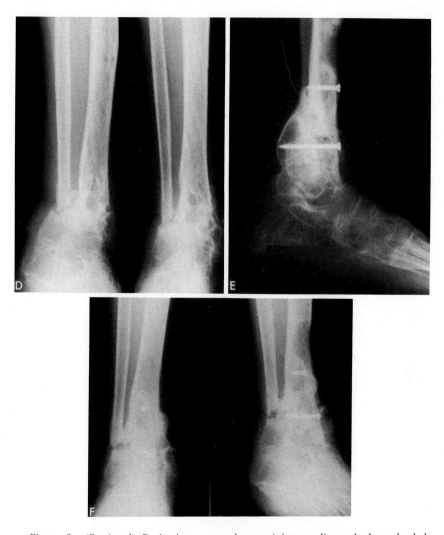

Figure 3. (*Continued*). *D*, At sixteen months post injury, radiograph shows healed soft tissue following sequestrectomy and nonunion of the tibia and fibula. *E* and *F*, Radiograph taken five months post-arthrodesis of the ankle with anterior sliding graph.

(*Figure 3 continued on the following page.*)

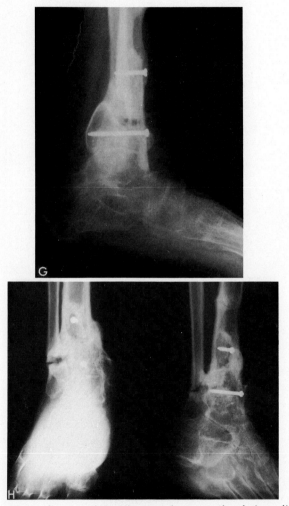

Figure 3 *(Continued)*.  *G* and *H*, Nine months post-arthrodesis, radiograph shows solid union of fracture of tibia and solid arthrodesis of ankle. There is valgus of foot and pain on prolonged weight bearing. The arthrodesis was classified as a poor result.

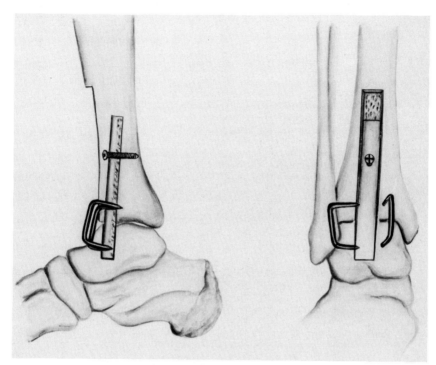

Figure 4. This is the technique of arthrodesis the authors prefer. In this series 58 per cent of the cases were performed by this technique or slight modification.

## REFERENCES

1. Adams, J. C.: Arthrodesis of the ankle. Experiences with a transfibular approach. J. Bone Joint Surg., *30B*:506-511, 1948.

2. Anderson, R.: Concentric arthrodesis of the ankle joint; transmalleolar approach. J. Bone Joint Surg., *27*:37-48, 1945.

3. Bagby, G. W.: Clinical experience of a simplified compression bone plate. Am. J. Orthop. Surg., *10*:302-311, 1968.

4. Baker, P. L.: SACH heel improves results of ankle fusion. J. Bone Joint Surg., *52A*:1485-1486, 1970.

5. Barr, J. S., and Record, E. E.: Arthrodesis of the ankle joint; indications, operative technic and clinical experience. N. Engl. J. Med., *248*:53-56, 1953.

6. Boyd, H. B.: Indications for fusion of the ankle. Orthop. Clin. North Am., *5*:191-192, 1974.

7. Brittain, H. A.: Architectural Principles in Arthrodesis. Edition 2. Edinburgh, E. S. Livingstone Ltd., 1952, pp. 1-20, 105-111.

8. Brooks, A. L., and Saunders, E. H.: Fusion of the ankle in denervated extremities. South. Med. J., *60*:30-33, 1967.

9. Broomhead, R., et al.: Discussion on fractures in region of ankle joint. Proc. Roy. Soc. Med., *25*:1082-1097, 1932.

10. Campbell, C. J., Rinehart, W. T., and Kalenak, A.: Arthrodesis of the ankle; deep autologous inlay grafts with maximum cancellous-bone apposition. J. Bone Joint Surg., *56A*:63-70, 1974.

11. Campbell, W. C.: Operation for induction of osseous fusion in the ankle joint. Am. J. Surg., *6*:588-592, 1929.

12. Charnley, J.: Ankle fusion in severe paralytic deformities of the foot. *In* Charnley, J.: Compression Arthrodesis. London, E. S. Livingstone, Ltd., 1953, pp. 157-164.

13. Charnley, J.: Compression arthrodesis of the ankle. *In* Charnley, J.: Compression Arthrodesis. London, E. S. Livingstone, Ltd., 1953, pp. 133-156.

14. Chuinard, E. G., and Peterson, R. E.: Distraction-compression bone graft arthrodesis of the ankle. A method especially applicable in children. J. Bone Joint Surg., 45A:481-490, 1963.

15. Cordebar, J.: Reconstitution of the tibia-tarsal joint. Presse Med., 64:1774, 1956.

16. Crenshaw, A. H. (Editor): Arthrodesis. *In* Campbell's Operative Orthopaedics. Edition 5. St. Louis, C. V. Mosby Co., 1971, pp. 1125-1134.

17. Fjermeros, H., and Hagen, R.: Post-traumatic arthrosis in the ankle and foot treated with arthrodesis. Acta Chir. Scand., 133:527-532, 1967.

18. Gallie, W. E.: Arthrodesis of ankle joint. J. Bone Joint Surg., 30B:619-621, 1948.

19. Giberson, R. G., and Janes, J. M.: Tibiocalcaneal fusion; surgical technique. Surg. Gynecol. Obstet., 99:773-776, 1954.

20. Glissan, D. J.: Indications for inducing fusion at ankle joint by operation, with description of two successful techniques. Aust. N.Z.J. Surg., 19:64-71, 1949.

21. Graham, C. E.: A new method for arthrodesis of an ankle joint. Clin. Orthop., 68:75-77, 1970.

22. Hallock, H.: Arthrodesis of ankle joint for old painful fractures. J. Bone Joint Surg., 27:49-58, 1945.

23. Hellstadius, A.: Apparatus for firm apposition of resectional surfaces in intra-articular arthrodesis. Acta Orthop. Scand., 11:190-198, 1940.

24. Hone, M. R.: Dowel fusion of the ankle joint. J. Bone Joint Surg., 50B:678, 1968.

25. Horwitz, T.: Use of the transfibular approach in arthrodesis of ankle joint. Am. J. Surg., 55:550-552, 1942.

26. Jansen, K.: Arthrodesis of the ankle joint. Acta Orthop. Scand., 32:476-484, 1962.

27. Johnson, E. W., Jr., and Boseker, E. H.: Arthrodesis of the ankle. Arch. Surg., 97:766-773, 1968.

28. Karlen, A.: On arthrodesis of the ankle joint in post traumatic conditions. Acta Orthop. Scand., 18:175-185, 1948.

29. Kennedy, J. C.: Arthrodesis of the ankle joint with particular reference to the Gallie procedure; a review of fifty cases. J. Bone Joint Surg., 42A:1308-1316, 1960.

30. Kimberley, A. G.: Malunited fractures affecting ankle joint, with special reference to 22 cases treated by arthrodesis. Surg. Gynecol. Obstet., 62:79-84, 1936.

31. Kivilaakso, R., Langenskiold, A., and Salenius, P.: Arthrodesis of the ankle as a treatment for post-fracture conditions. Acta Orthop. Scand., 37:409-414, 1966.

32. Kovanda, M., and Muller, I.: Arthrodesis of the upper talar articulation in post-traumatic conditions. Acta Chir. Orthop. Traumatol. Cech., 39:370-372, 1972.

33. Liebolt, F. L.: Pantalar arthrodesis in poliomyelitis. Surgery, 6:31-34, 1939.

34. Lukasik, S.: Distraction compression arthrodesis of the ankle joint with the use of a bone graft stored at low temperature. Bull. Pol. Med. Sci. Hist., 10:72-75, 1967.

35. Mead, N. C.: Arthrodesis of ankle joint; simple, efficient method. Q. Bull. Northwest Univ. School Med., 25:248-250, 1951.

36. Miller, J. W.: Coarse threaded screw internal fixation as an adjunct to ankle joint fusion. Bull. Mason Clin., 14:138-144, 1960.

37. Morris, H. D.: Arthrodesis of the foot. Clin. Orthop., 16:164-176, 1960.

38. Morris, H. D.: Aseptic necrosis of the talus following injury. Orthop. Clin. North Am., 5:177-189, 1974.

39. Morris. H. D., Hand, W. L., and Dunn, A. W.: The modified Blair fusion for fractures of the talus. J. Bone Joint Surg., 53A:1289-1297, 1971.

40. Ottolenghi, C. E., Animoso, J., and Burgo, P. H.: Percutaneous arthrodesis of the ankle joint. Clin. Orthop., 68:72-74, 1970.

41. Pridie, K. H.: Arthrodesis of the ankle. J. Bone Joint Surg., 35B:152, 1953.

42. Ratliff, A. H.: Compression arthrodesis of the ankle. J. Bone Joint Surg., 41B:524-534, 1959.

43. Sammarco, G. J., Burstein, A. H., and Frankel, V. H.: Biomechanics of the ankle joint: A kinematic study. Orthop. Clin. North Am., 4:75-96, 1973.

44. Sharp, N., et al.: Ankle fusions in children. J. Bone Joint Surg., 45A:1549, 1963.

45. Soren, A.: Safe inlay of bone graft in arthrodesis. Clin. Orthop., *58*:147-152, 1968.

46. Soulies A., et al.: Tibiotarsal arthrodesis using cylindrical grafts. Acta Orthop. Belg., *35*:377-391, 1969.

47. Speed, J. S., and Boyd, H. B.: Operative reconstruction of malunited fractures about ankle joint. J. Bone Joint Surg., *18*:270-286, 1936.

48. Thomas, F. B.: Arthrodesis at the ankle. J. Bone Joint Surg., *51B*:53-59, 1969.

49. Vahvanen, V.: Arthrodesis of the TC or pantalar joints in rheumatoid arthritis. Acta Orthop. Scand., *40*:642-652, 1969.

50. Vahvanen, V., and Rokkanen, P.: Arthrodesis of the ankle. Ann. Chir. Gyanecol. Fenn., *61*:37-40, 1972.

51. Vainio, S.: Arthrodesis of the ankle in the treatment of a malunited fracture. Ann. Chir. Gyanecol. Fenn., *46* (Suppl. 69):1-37, 1957.

52. Wang, C. J., Tambakis, A. P., and Fielding, J. W.: An evaluation of ankle fusion in children. Clin. Orthop., *98*:233-238, 1974.

53. Wescott, H. H.: An operation for the fusion of the tibio-astragaloid joint. Va. Med. Mon., *61*:38-39, 1934.

54. White, A. A., III: A precision posterior ankle fusion. Clin. Orthop., *98*:239-250, 1974.

55. Wilson, H. J., Jr.: Arthrodesis of the ankle; a technique using bilateral hemimalleolar onlay grafts with screw fixation. J. Bone Joint Surg., *51A*:775-777, 1969.

*Chapter 10*

# Anterior Dowel Fusion
# of the Ankle

CHARLES F. HEINIG, M.D.*

DAVID N. DUPUY, M.D.†

In the past, more than 20 different methods have been described to solve the problem of a painful, unstable, or diseased ankle. These include approaches from all conceivable angles and various types of fixation. None has been universally acceptable to the orthopedic surgeon. This is why in 1972, White[26] entitled his exhibit at the Academy, "And Yet Another Ankle Fusion."

To be universally acceptable, the operation must be simple and safe and yet have a high fusion rate; it must be applicable to the old and the young; and it must have a low morbidity and heal rapidly. Gallie[7] wrote in 1948, "that probably his excuse for presenting his method was that as we grow older we seek easier ways of doing our operations, and more certain methods of protecting our reputations by lessening the risk of failure."

Johnson and Boseker,[16] in 1968, reported on 140 fusions in 132 patients, using various methods and approaches, noting 84 complications or a 60 per cent incidence. Fortunately most were minor, however 21 patients had sepsis, five had pseudarthrosis, 11 had chronic foot and ankle swelling, 10 had delayed wound healing, seven had significant post arthrosis pain, and six patients required amputation. Their comment was "this series demonstrates that the greater the scope of the operation about the ankle, the less the chances of success." They did not feel that iliac crest graft gave satisfactory end results in their cases. Reports such as this have prompted many of us to look for newer and better methods.

Ottolenghi,[19] for example, described a percutaneous arthrodesis of the ankle joint in 1968, in an attempt to obtain fusion with minimal trauma. Charnley[5] popularized compression arthrodesis. He laid the ankle joint open anteriorly, and cut all the tendons, dorsalis pedis artery, and the nerves to the dorsum of the foot. He denuded the ankle sur-

---

* Chairman, Department of Orthopaedic Surgery, Charlotte Memorial Hospital and Medical Center, Charlotte, North Carolina.
† Senior Orthopedic Resident, Charlotte Memorial Hospital and Medical Center, Charlotte, North Carolina.

150

faces, placed them in the desired position, compressed them for four weeks with compression clamps, and supported the soft tissues with bandages while they healed. At four weeks, dressings and pins were removed and a cast was applied for an additional four weeks. At the end of the eight weeks, all immobilization was removed, regardless of what x-ray films showed. In his first 19 cases, four had fibrous ankylosis and one had subtalar and midtalar pain. Ratliff[21] later reported on this series of patients stating that 50 per cent of the 55 needlessly wore casts for 12 to 14 weeks. There had been no evidence of circulation problems following the cutting of the dorsalis pedis artery and most people did not complain about the 50 per cent loss of toe motion nor the loss of sensation over the dorsum of the foot.

We were confronted with some patients in whom trauma had been so severe that the foot and leg had been considered to be in jeopardy for many days. We decided to modify the Gallie operation by using dowels of cancellous iliac bone rather than cortical strut grafts from the tibia. It was felt that the foot and ankle could be stabilized in the desired position by being jigged with a large Steinmann pin, which was driven up through the os calcis and subtalar joint into the ankle joint (Fig. 1, *A* and *B*).

## OPERATIVE PROCEDURE

With the ankle stabilized with the Steinmann pin in desired position of 0 to a maximum of 5 degrees of equinus, the operative procedure begins by making two small anterior incisions, one medially and one laterally, curvilinear in nature. Each of the incisions begins at the tip of its respective malleolus and courses in an arched manner toward the midline, leaving approximately 1½ inches of skin over the tendons and dorsalis pedis area (Fig. 1C). The medial side of the ankle is exposed first, removing the soft tissues and synovium. The front of the talus and the medial malleolus and plafond are then squared off with an osteotome and a gouge in such a manner that a ½ inch dowel cutter may be inserted along the medial portion of the medial malleolus, the dome of the talus, and the medial surface of the plafond of the tibia. Using a hand chuck or T wrench, a ½ inch dowel cutter is used (Fig. 1D). Care is taken to leave the back of the ankle joint intact to protect its vital structures. By using a ¼ inch slightly curved osteotome, it is possible to remove the doweled area, which includes the joint line, with ease. Similarly, the ankle joint is exposed laterally and after removal of soft tissue the fibula, part of the tibia, and talus are squared off with an osteotome and a gouge, again to receive the ½ inch dowel cutter, which now cuts a dowel from the top of the tibia and lateral malleolus and the dome of the talus. Care is used to protect the posterior integrity of the ankle joint and the dowel is removed.

Usually fragments of cartilage and bone removed are not used in the fusion except in persons with rheumatoid arthritis. The cartilage does not have to be removed from the joint surface. In fact, it helps to maintain

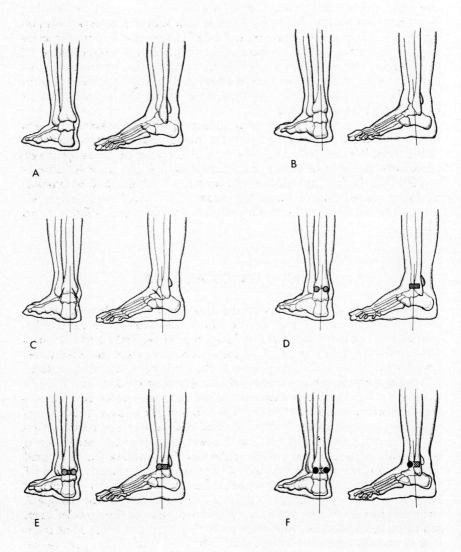

Figure 1. Operative procedure for anterior dowel fusion of the ankle. *A*, Position foot in 0 to 5 degrees of equinus. *B*, Insert the Steinmann pin blindly. *C*, Make two anterior incisions. *D*, Cut the medial and lateral dowels ½ inch in diameter and insert ⅝ inch dowels from iliac crest. *E*, A third dowel may be taken anteriorly, but is not necessary and may increase instability of the ankle. *F*, Insert three ⅝ inch dowels and put on a soft compression dressing with pin in place.

the height and stability of the ankle if left in place. As Gallie has noted, and we concur, the cartilage eventually incorporates in the fusion. If the ankle has been crushed particularly anteriorly and the surgeon wishes to denude a greater surface of the tibia and talus, a third dowel may be taken anteriorly to the pin directed from the lateral surface in front of the fibula and directed toward the medial malleolus (Fig. 1E). This encompasses the dome of the talus anteriorly in the anterior aspect of the tibial plafond. Unfortunately this tends to make the ankle more unstable and may interfere with branches of the dorsalis pedis artery through the talus, as well as branches of the artery from the tarsal canal and the deltoid branches of the posterior tibial artery.

Next, a ⅝ inch dowel is taken from anterior to posterior along the very top of the crest, beginning at the anterior superior iliac spine. We take both the inner and outer tables for a distance of approximately 5 to 6 cm., which is adequate to replace the two or three dowels that have been taken from the ankle joint. A ⅝ inch dowel of bone will fill a ½ inch hole very snugly and is driven against the back of the ankle mortice. Any little fragments of bone that are available may be used to fill up the voids (Fig. 1F). As previously noted, the ankle surfaces do not need to be denuded, but if the surgeon wishes, there is no reason not to do it.

Wounds are closed with a subcuticular Dexon closure, which aids skin healing. The patient is quite comfortable in a soft dressing with the pin extending through the os calcis, talus, and into the tibia.

At approximately the tenth postoperative day, the soft bulky dressing is removed if the ankle mortice is felt to be stable, and in the two dowel fusion the pin may be removed and a short leg walking cast applied The patient is allowed to bear weight as soon as he desires. If a third anterior dowel has been taken and the ankle appears somewhat unstable, it is advisable to leave the pin in place for at least six weeks. The minimal time of immobilization is 12 to 14 weeks. Here, clinical judgment must enter into any surgical procedure. We have erred at least on two occasions because of early enthusiasm to remove fixation at 11 to 12 weeks, when, in fact, healing was not adequate. It is difficult to determine complete healing because the circulation to the talus is the secret to healing of an ankle fusion. It takes about six to eight months for the trabecular pattern to become apparent and probably a year for healing to become complete. Several cases are presented to demonstrate the rate of healing.

### Results

Because of considerable pain postoperatively, it was essential to re-explore one of our fusions. Opinions from other physicians as well as a laminogram, indicated pseudarthrosis. At the exploration, the ankle joint was found to be solid. Subsequent laminograms taken postoperatively, showed that the fusion was solid by laminogram and that the subtalar joint was arthritic. With severe trauma seen in motor vehicle accidents, particularly motorcycles, trauma to many joints may be the rule rather than the exception. For this reason it is often difficult after severe and multiple injuries to determine which patients will benefit most from ankle fusion.

Two patients developed pseudarthrosis because they were removed from plaster immobilization at 12 weeks. Clinically, these were not solid. One patient developed a wound infection and the skin over both malleoli sloughed, requiring a skin graft. The skin between the malleoli anteriorly remained intact. Grafting was carried out while the ankle was stabilized with a pin. Solid fusion ensued and the skin grafts were successful.

## DISCUSSION

Our observations indicate that the foot should be placed in 0 to 5 degrees of equinus. Care should be used in selecting patients for fusion in whom there are other arthritic joints. The extent of subtalar involvement is difficult to assess. Patients have difficulty in separating the origin of pain in these two joints.

## SUMMARY

A modified anterior Gallie fusion of the ankle has been carried out in 18 patients, 17 were of traumatic origin and one rheumatoid arthritis; of these two cases of pseudarthrosis developed. Two patients have continued to have some discomfort, with a minor limp caused by subtalar arthritis. One patient developed skin loss over the malleoli but satisfactory bony union occurred. The method is not applicable for correction of bony deformity. We have not used it in children, but see no reason that it could not be safely and easily carried out because it does not involve the epiphysis and there is no loss of height.

## REFERENCES

1. Adams, J. C.: Arthrodesis of the ankle joint. J. Bone Joint Surg., 30B:506-511, 1948.

2. Anderson, R.: Concentric arthrodesis of the ankle joint. J. Bone Joint Surg., 27:37, 1945.

3. Barr, J. S., and Record, E. E.: Arthrodesis of the ankle joint. Indications, operative technique and clinical experience. New Eng. J. Med., 248:53-56, 1953.

4. Bingold, A. C.: Ankle and subtalar fusion by a transarticular graft. J. Bone Joint Surg., 38B:862-870, 1956.

5. Charnley, J.: Compression arthrodesis of the ankle and shoulder. J. Bone Joint Surg., 33B:180-191, 1951.

6. Chuinard, E. G., and Peterson, R. E.: Distraction-compression bone graft arthrodesis of the ankle. A method especially applicable in children. J. Bone Joint Surg., 45A:481-490, 1963.

7. Gallie, W. E.: Arthrodesis of the ankle joint. J. Bone Joint Surg., 30B:619-621, 1948.

8. Goldthwait, J. E.: An operation for the stiffening of the ankle joint in infantile paralysis. Amer. J. Orthop. Surg., 5:271-275, 1907-1908.

9. Graham, C. E.: A new method for arthrodesis of an ankle joint. Clin. Orthop., 68:75-77, 1970.

10. Hallock, H.: Arthrodesis of the ankle joint for old painful fractures. J. Bone Joint Surg., 27:49-58, 1945.

11. Hatt, R. N.: The central bone graft in joint arthrodesis. J. Bone Joint Surg., 22:393-402, 1940.

12. Hone, M. R.:Dowel fusion of the ankle joint. J. Bone Joint Surg., 50B:678, 1968.

13. Horowitz, T.: The use of the transfibular approach in arthrodesis of the ankle joint. Am. J. Surg., 55:550-552, 1942.

14. Hurley, L. A., Zeier, F. G., and Stinchfield, F. E.: Anorganic bone grafting. Am. J. Surg., 101:12-21, 1960.

15. Jansen, K.: Arthrodesis of the ankle joint. Acta Orthop. Scand., 32:476-484, 1962.

16. Johnson, E. W., and Boseker, E. H.: Arthrodesis of the ankle. Arch. Surg., 97:766-773, 1968.

17. Kennedy, J. C.: Arthrodesis of the ankle with particular reference to the Gallie procedure. A review of fifty cases. J. Bone Joint Surg., 42A:1308-1316, 1960.

18. Mulfinger, G. L., and Treuta, J.: The blood supply of the talus. J. Bone Joint Surg., 52B:160-167, 1970.

19. Ottolenghi, C. E., Animoso, J., and Burgo, P. H.: Percutaneous arthrodesis of the ankle joint. Clin. Orthop., 68:72-74, 1970.

20. Pridie, K. H.: Arthrodesis of the ankle. J. Bone Joint Surg., 35B:152, 1953.

21. Ratliff, A. H. C.: Compression arthrodesis of the ankle. J. Bone Joint Surg., 41B:524-534, 1959.

22. Soren, A.: Safe inlay of bone graft in arthrodesis. Clin. Orthop., 58:147-152, 1968.

23. Staples, S. O.: Posterior arthrodesis of the ankle and the subtalar joints. J. Bone Joint Surg., 38A:50-58, 1956.

24. Thomas, F. B.: Arthrodesis of the ankle. J. Bone Joint Surg., 51B:53-59, 1969.

25. Watson-Jones, R.: Fractures and Joint Injuries. Edition 4, Vol. 2, Baltimore, Williams and Wilkins Co. 1956, p. 854.

26. White, A. A., and Hirsch, C.: An experimental study of the immediate load bearing capacity of some commonly used iliac bone grafts. Acta Orthop. Scand., 42:482-490, 1971.

27. Wilson, H.: Arthrodesis of the ankle. A technique using bilateral hemimalleolar only grafts with screw fixation. J. Bone Joint Surg., 51A:775-777, 1969.

*Chapter 11*

# Arthrodesis of the Ankle

JOHN R. HUCKELL, M.D.C.M., F.R.C.S.(C)*

JOHN FULLER, M.B.Ch.B., F.R.C.S.(C)†

"Arthrodesis is an effective means of relieving the pain and disability that often arise from old ankle fractures." This was the conclusion of Hallock,[5] in 1945, who studied the results of arthrodesis in 39 patients, and recommended a position of fusion in 10 degrees of equinus. Since that time experience has cast doubt on the efficacy of ankle fusion, especially in the equinus position. There have only been a few clinical studies of arthrodesis. Kimberley,[6] in 1936, recommended arthrodesis as a salvage procedure after malunion of fractures about the ankle. In 1948, Adams[1] reviewed 30 cases of ankle fusion using the transfibular approach. Barr and Record,[2] in 1953, reviewed the results of arthrodesis in 50 patients. In 1959, Ratliff reported 50 cases of compression arthrodesis, and suggested that the optimal position for fusion was in neutral, at or close to a right angle. Dewar,[4] in 1971, studied 50 cases of ankle fusion following closed fractures about the ankle.

Most authors stress that this is not a common procedure, and is performed for the more severe cases where conservative measures have failed. The aim of this study is to ascertain how effective fusion of the ankle is in meeting the demands of severe cases, and the effect of technique and the position of fusion on the functional result.

## CLINICAL MATERIAL

There were 45 ankle fusions performed by the staff of the University of Alberta Hospital between 1962 and 1972. Twenty-eight patients were traced and replied to a questionnaire; of these 20 were examined clinically. The shortest period of observation was one year and the longest 10 years. The age of the patients at the time of observation varied from 19 to 65, with the majority between 40 and 60 years. Nineteen were male and nine female, but in those fused for traumatic arthritis, 16 were male and four female.

---

* Assistant Clinical Professor, University of Alberta, Edmonton, Alberta, Canada.
† Active Staff, Surrey Memorial Hospital, Surrey, British Columbia, Canada.

The conditions for which arthrodesis were performed were in the majority traumatic arthritis and poliomyelitis. Twenty of the 28 fusions were performed for degenerative arthritis with pain following fractures around the ankle. This included closed, open, and multiple fractures. The time between injury and fusion varied from immediately after to 35 years following fracture.

The techniques used to achieve fusion were varied. The most common technique, used in 10 patients, was fibular onlay. In seven patients the joint space was packed with cancellous chips and the position maintained by a Kirschner wire passing vertically through the joint. A sliding bone graft from the tibia was used in six patients, compression arthrodesis in four patients, and the Gallie technique in one patient.

Five patients required a second attempt at fusion. Failure of arthrodesis occurred in four patients in whom bone chips were used, and in one fibular onlay graft. Packing with bone chips appears to be an inferior technique.

## RESULTS

### Subjective

Fourteen of the 28 patients, that is half of those traced, were pleased with the result. Nineteen have pain. Twenty-three complained of a limp; of these eight used a cane and four a heel lift (Fig. 1). Seventeen were able to function as well as they wished at home. Only three men and two women were able to do the type of work they were doing before injury without restriction. Three men worked with pain and restriction, and one man was retired. Only two did not feel restricted in their recreation.

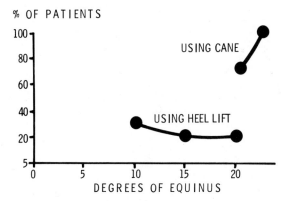

Figure 1.  Twenty-three of the 28 patients followed complained of a limp; of these eight used a cane and four used a heel lift.

### Objective

Of the 20 patients examined none had a normal gait barefoot. Seven had a normal gait when wearing shoes. Two were unable to walk barefoot. Two patients were unable to walk due to their basic preoperative condition, one had had severe poliomyelitis, the other had progressive rheumatoid arthritis.

There were four main problems in gait, the chief of which were hyperextension of the knee and pain in the forefoot with motion due to arthrodesis in a position of excessive equinus. In the patients with hyperextension of the knee and forefoot pain, six had both, three had hyperextension alone, and one had forefoot pain alone. The later had excessive equinus corrected. Two women and nine men were fused in less than 15 degrees of equinus, whereas five women and four men were fused in more than 15 degrees of equinus.

### Complications

Three patients developed infections postoperatively; the initial infecting organism in two was Staphylococcus albus and in the other Staphylococcus aureus. One patient developed thrombophlebitis. Fusion was solid in all but two patients examined. One patient had diabetic neuropathic arthropathy; he developed pseudoarthrosis with discomfort he was willing to tolerate. The second patient developed painful pseudoarthrosis. Two patients required revision of fusion, and two required tibial osteotomy for malposition of the ankle. The unacceptable position giving rise to gait problems in these ankles was excessive equinus in three and calcaneovarus in one.

### Relationship of Function to Position of Fusion

Arthrodesis was performed in equinus to a varying extent, the commonest position being 10 degrees of equinus (Fig. 2). The problems

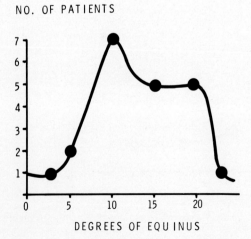

NO. OF PATIENTS

DEGREES OF EQUINUS

Figure 2. Varying degrees of equinus in which arthrodesis was carried out, 10 degrees being the most common.

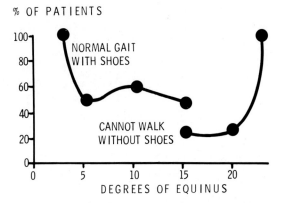

Figure 3.   Those patients with a normal gait while wearing shoes had an arthrodesis in a position of neutral to 15 degrees of equinus, whereas those who could not walk without shoes had a fusion in 15 degrees of equinus or more.

of gait were related to the degree of equinus. The quality of gait was similarly related to equinus. Those patients with a normal gait while wearing shoes had an arthrodesis in a position of neutral to 15 degrees of equinus, whereas those who could not walk without shoes had a fusion in fifteen degrees of equinus or more (Fig.3). One patient's ankle was fused in the neutral position did not have a normal gait; however, this was the patient who was managing with pseudoarthrosis following attempted fusion for neuropathic arthropathy.

Hyperextension of the knee was closely related to the degree of equinus, and its incidence increased with a greater degree of equinus. At 10 degrees of equinus two of seven patients experienced pain because of hyperextension; at 20 degrees three of four experienced pain (Fig.4).

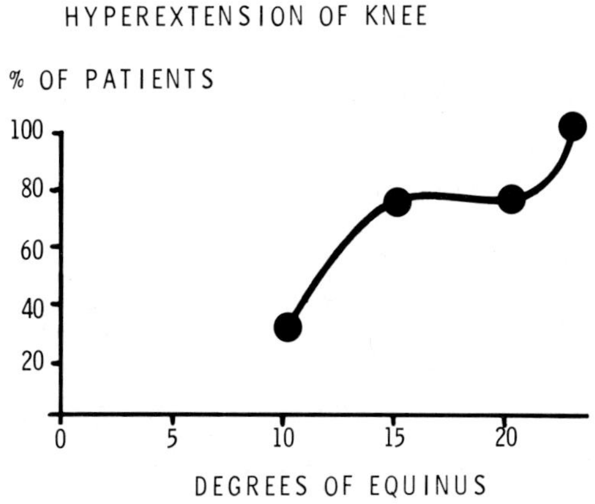

HYPEREXTENSION OF KNEE

% OF PATIENTS

```
100 ┤                                    ●
 80 ┤                    ●        ●
 60 ┤                 
 40 ┤            ●
 20 ┤
  0 └──┬────┬────┬────┬────
     0    5   10   15   20
       DEGREES OF EQUINUS
```

Figure 4.   Relationship of hyperextension of the knee to degree of equinus.

Forefoot pain was caused by abnormal weight bearing stresses forcing the forefoot into dorsiflexion, a movement normally occurring at the ankle joint. Forefoot pain was again closely related to the degree of equinus. It did not occur at less than 15 degrees of equinus where two of four patients experienced pain; at 20 degrees of equinus three of four patients had pain in the forefoot (Fig. 5). One patient who had a revision of ankle arthrodesis for excessive equinus continued to have metatarsalgia following correction, and also developed heel pain on weight bearing following correction.

The problem of callous formation beneath the metatarsal heads was similarly related to equinus. The incidence of patients requiring a heel lift or cane was increased with greater degrees of equinus. Heel pain did not appear to have any apparent relationship to the position of fusion. Lesser degrees of valgus or varus were noticed in some patients but were not found to have a marked bearing on function.

## DISCUSSION

This study has been based on 45 patients who underwent ankle arthrodesis, of whom 28 were traced and 20 examined. This has not been a common procedure in Edmonton and does not appear to be a desirable one. If fusion is performed, then the best position for the ankle is in neutral position, as suggested by Ratliff[7] in 1959. If a few degrees of equinus is desired when the ankle is fused in neutral position, this can be achieved by the more normal motion of plantar flexion at the tarsal joints. The results of this series have been poor enough for us to consider that the development of an alternative procedure is justified. The higher incidence of ankle fusion in the 50 to 60 year age group suggests that the development of a total ankle arthroplasty would be worthy of consideration.

Dewar in 1971 noted that "ankle fusion is associated with considera-

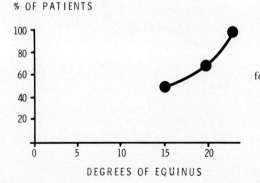

FOREFOOT PAIN WITH MOTION

% OF PATIENTS

Figure 5. Relationship of forefoot pain to degree of equinus.

DEGREES OF EQUINUS

ble morbidity and disability and should not be undertaken in desperation in the psychologically unstable patient. It is a very useful salvage procedure in an area where joint reconstruction or replacement has not yet been developed."

## REFERENCES

1. Adams, J. C.: Arthrodesis of the ankle joint. Experiences with the transfibular approach. J. Bone Joint Surg., *30B*:506, 1948.
2. Barr, J. S., and Record, E. E.: Arthrodesis of the ankle joint. Indications, operative technique and clinical experience. New Eng. J. Med., *245*:53, 1953.
3. Charnley, J.: Compression arthrodesis of the ankle and shoulder. J. Bone Joint Surg., *33B*:180, 1951.
4. Dewar, F. P., and Martin, F. R.: Ankle fusions following closed ankle fractures. J. Bone Joint Surg., *54B*:768, 1972.
5. Hallock, H.: Arthrodesis of the ankle joint for old painful fractures. J. Bone Joint Surg., *27*:49, 1945.
6. Kimberley, A. G.: Malunited fractures affecting the ankle joint. Surg. Gynecol. Obstet. *62*:79, 1936.
7. Ratliff, A. H.: Compression arthrodesis of the ankle. J. Bone Joint Surg., *41B*:524, 1959.

*Chapter 12*

# Talectomy

RICHARD M. KILFOYLE, M.D.*

JAMES S. BROOME, M.D.†

JAMES H. HARDY, M.D.‡

BURR H. CURTIS, M.D.§

Talectomy is not a new procedure, having enjoyed a long period of popularity followed by a long period of disrepute and disuse. Despite its acceptance in many quarters as an operation designed to correct deformities of the foot, particularly calcaneus and calcaneoval-gus deformities, many orthopedic surgeons refuse to consider its occasional use for any indication other than those named. Their objections to removal of the talus are well taken: the length and height of the foot are reduced, correspondingly the malleoli are lowered rendering shoe-fitting difficult especially in women; and degenerative arthritis of the tibiocalcaneal articulation sometimes develops in later years necessitating a fusion — an operation that is not always successful. Notwithstanding these very relevant objections, there remains a select group of young patients with rigid deformity, whose need to have plantigrade feet can probably not be satisfied by other means. They are too young for triple arthrodesis and some have deformities which cannot be well corrected by this procedure. In fact, the members of this relatively small group represent failures of more conventional treatment such as manipulation, stretching, serial casting, and operative soft tissue procedures, such as medial releases, capsulotomies, tendon releases or transfers. Radical and unphysiological as it seems, talectomy is offered as a solution to the problem of the severe rigid deformed foot in the young child. Children with severe, uncorrected rigid deformities preventing a plantigrade

* Clinical Professor of Orthopedic Surgery and Fractures, Boston University School of Medicine, Boston, Massachusetts.
† Instructor in Orthopedics, Tufts University School of Medicine, Boston, Massachusetts; Chief of Orthopedics, USPHS Hospital, Brighton, Massachusetts.
‡ Clinical Assistant Professor of Orthopedic Surgery, University of Connecticut Medical Center, Farmington, Connecticut.
§ Clinical Professor of Orthopedics, Department of Surgery, University of Connecticut Medical Center, Farmington; Medical and Executive Director, Newington Children's Hospital, Newington, Connecticut.

posture of the foot have little available to them except supracondylar osteotomies or watchful waiting until the age for arthrodesis has been reached.

## HISTORY

The first recorded talectomy was done by Fabricus of Hilden in 1608 for an open fracture and, until 1899, open fracture and local disease of the talus were the only generally accepted indications for the procedure. In 1901, Royal Whitman[5] reported the first of his several papers on the treatment of paralytic talipes of the calcaneal type. Thompson[4] in 1939 reviewed Whitman's results in over 2000 recorded cases. After personal inspection of many of the longterm follow-ups, he reaffirmed its usefulness. Another evaluation of talectomy by O'Donoghue[2] in 1956 favored restriction of the operation to Whitman's original narrow indications; however O'Donoghue did note successful reports of talectomy in severe, congenital clubfoot and arthrogryposis. It remained for Sharrard[3] in 1968 and Menelaus[1] in 1971 to give well documented sanction for talectomy in rigid equinovarus deformities secondary to arthrogryposis and spina bifida.

## MATERIAL

Most of our cases involved correction of severe deformities in children with myelomeningocele and arthrogryposis. Two patients underwent talectomy for correction of relapsed clubfoot. One patient had severe equinovarus deformities associated with a chondrodystrophy. Another patient with multiple congenital anomalies of the right foot underwent the operation. We have not treated any patients with convex pes valgus by talectomy. There are 10 patients in our series ranging in age from 10 months to 10 years (the patient with the chondrodystrophy) at the time of operation, an age range in which arthrodesing procedures are not advisable. The median age is seven years. Ten patients underwent a total of 12 talectomies. There were 35 pretalectomy surgical procedures performed on the feet of these 10 patients.

## OPERATIVE TECHNIQUE

Talectomy is a relatively simple procedure and our technique differs little from the standard method. A few points deserve repeated emphasis. It is imperative to displace the foot posteriorly far enough so that the tip of the fibula reaches the calcaneocuboid joint level with the medial malleolus just above and behind the navicular. This displacement of the calcaneus provides a long lever arm which gives a mechanical advantage to the calf muscles. The foot should not be aligned with the patella, but should be externally rotated beneath the leg. This is the stable position for the new articulation. In order to obtain this stable status, we do not hesitate to divide the tendo Achilles and the inferior-most fibers of the tibiofibular ligaments. Internal fixation of the foot to the tibia can be carried out by the use of one or two Steinmann pins which traverse the calcaneus and enter the tibia.

Plaster fixation, or pin fixation, or both should be maintained for a period of six to eight weeks after which walking is allowed.

## CLINICAL EXPERIENCE

CASE 1.   A. M., a nine year old boy, presented with arthrogryposis multiplex congenita. As in all our patients, our aim was to give this boy well aligned, stable joints for independent locomotion. He came to us from another state hospital where he had undergone multiple operative procedures on the lower extremities. As an infant, he had heel cord lengthenings and, more recently, had extensive medial releases of both feet. He sloughed a large portion of the medial aspect of his right foot following the medial release and the deformity remained uncorrected. Before attempting talectomy, good skin and soft tissue covering of his foot were obtained by a cross-leg pedicle flap. Later, in June 1973, he underwent talectomy to correct the rigid equinovarus foot. The illustrations indicate that before talectomy the patient had the characteristic elfin or wooden doll appearance of arthrogryposis and multiple congenital flexion deformities of multiple joints. He also had diminished muscle substance with the characteristic appearance of wasting. As previously noted there is decreased active and passive range of motion of his joints, the normal skin creases are absent, and the skin is tense and glossy. After talectomy, a plantigrade foot was achieved.

CASE 2.   M. H., a five year old girl, presented with rigid equinus deformity of both feet with flat-top talus (Fig. 1). The persistent equinus was a result of congenital hypoplasia of all muscles below the knees. By far, the strongest of these was the gastrocnemius soleus. She had abduction of the right forefoot and adduction of the left. Previously, at the age of one, she had Achilles tendon sections percutaneously. She subsequently had lengthenings and posterior capsulotomies. Later in an attempt to balance the muscle pull this procedure was carried out: transfer on the right side of the medial half of the tendo Achilles to the mid-dorsum of the foot around the medial side of the tibia was accompanied by lengthening of the remaining half; on the left foot, the same procedure was carried out passing the divided tendon through the interosseous septum again to the mid-dorsum. These procedures had worked well for a short time but the deformity recurred, persisted, and became rigid, with flattening of the dome of the talus. At the age of four, she had a medial release with some improvement of the right foot. Early in her fifth year, in 1973, she underwent bilateral talectomy as a desperate measure. This was made imperative by progressing back knee deformity on both sides.

While most of her skeletal deformities are clustered around her feet and ankles, and while she has little other in the way of deformity in her uppermost extremities, we feel she represents a child with arthrogryposis. Her resistant equinus was perhaps simply a manifestation of this underlying disease state in the presence of muscle imbalance.

CASE 3.   L. M. was the first patient to have a talectomy in this series (Fig. 2). She came to us (from another state hospital) with the multiple deformities of chondrodystrophy. She had severe flexion deformities of both hips and knees

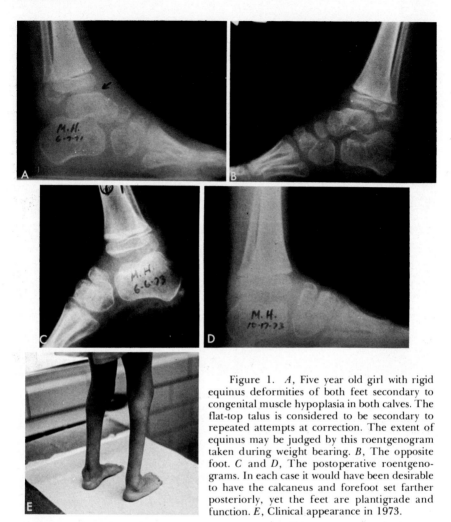

Figure 1. *A*, Five year old girl with rigid equinus deformities of both feet secondary to congenital muscle hypoplasia in both calves. The flat-top talus is considered to be secondary to repeated attempts at correction. The extent of equinus may be judged by this roentgenogram taken during weight bearing. *B*, The opposite foot. *C* and *D*, The postoperative roentgenograms. In each case it would have been desirable to have the calcaneus and forefoot set farther posteriorly, yet the feet are plantigrade and function. *E*, Clinical appearance in 1973.

accompanied by severe, rigid equinovarus deformities of both feet. The patient was able to walk with the aid of crutches, long leg braces, and special shoes; however the foot deformities became so severe, she was walking almost literally on her fifth toes. This became so painful that the ability to walk was jeopardized. At the age of 10, in 1959, she underwent bilateral talectomies with material improvement in the contour of both feet. She regained the ability to walk; she has retained that ability to this day, and supports herself as the manager of a busy answering service.

CASE 4.   The last patient is not one of our series, but is included to illustrate long term follow-up, with ultimate pain and the means of retrieving the situation in later life. W. S. is a 42 year old man who contracted polio as a child.

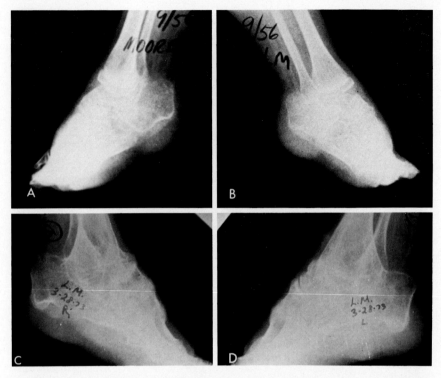

Figure 2. *A*, and *B*, Patient with chondrodystrophy—our first talectomy. The gross deformities may be judged by roentgenograms taken preoperatively. *C* and *D*, The postoperative appearance after a 14 year follow-up. Although the patient needs two long-leg braces and crutches, she walks well and manages an answering service.

He underwent talectomy at the age of eight. Thirty-four years later increasing pain required a tibiocalcaneal fusion which was carried out in 1973. He is currently back on his feet and walking well.

Another patient came to our attention and represents the longest follow-up of which we are personally aware. He was 92 years old and his talus was removed by Dr. E. H. Bradford 90 years before. His foot had served him well those 90 years until a wound infection resulted in death.

## CONCLUSION

None of these severely deformed children has normal feet. They are however able to walk with braces and crutches as needed. Their feet are plantigrade and they are able to wear shoes. We continue to reserve the use of talectomy for these extreme cases, almost desperate cases, and we regard it as being a valuable tool in our armamentarium.

# REFERENCES

1.   Menelaus, M. B.: Talectomy for equinovarus deformity in arthrogryposis and spina bifida. J. Bone Joint Surg., *53B*: 1971.

2. O'Donoghue, D. H.: An evaluation of astragalectomy. South Med. J., *49*:1128, 1956.

3. Sharrard, W. J. W.: The management of deformity and paralysis of the foot in myelomeningocele. J. Bone Joint Surg., *50B*:456, 1968.

4. Thompson, T. C.: Astragalectomy and the treatment of calcaneal valgus. J. Bone Joint Surg., *21*:627-647, 1939.

5. Whitman, R.: The operative treatment of paralytic talipes of the calcaneus type. Trans. Am. Orthop. Assoc. *14*:178, 1901.

# Chapter 13

# Talectomy for Osteomyelitis of the Talus

ALLEN W. JACKSON, M.D.*

ROBERT J. NEVIASER, M.D.†

JOHN P. ADAMS, M.D.‡

Injuries of the talus have been a serious and difficult problem for centuries. Fabricus[7] in 1608 reported the first talectomy for an open fracture. He was surprised at the good result. Cooper[5] in 1818 recommended talectomy for open fracture or dislocation of the talus. Syme[17] resorted to below-knee amputation for compound fracture-dislocation of the talus because of an 84 per cent mortality rate from infection in these injuries.

It was not until 1901 that Whitman[18] popularized talectomy. He showed that a useful and stable foot could be obtained when the procedure was performed properly and the patients were selected carefully. He recommended the procedure as a stabilizing operation for paralytic calcaneus and calcaneovalgus deformities in children between the ages of five and 15 years. The procedure gained wide acceptance and was used for virtually all deformities of the foot.[8] It became the accepted treatment for fracture-dislocation of the talus.[1, 16] Graham and Faulkner[8] reported on 10 talectomies for fracture, 70 per cent of which achieved satisfactory results. With the relaxation of Whitman's rigid criteria for talectomy there was an increase in the number of poor results.

With the control of poliomyelitis in our population, talectomy is now rarely performed. The procedure received mention in recent studies only to be condemned.[3, 12, 14] Miller and Baker[12] advocated arthrodesis for painful joints that may develop from a poor result after closed or open reduction of fractures of the talus. They advised against talectomy except in the presence of infection. Coltart[3] reported 228 major fractures of the talus from war injuries. Only 22 required excision

* Attending Orthopedic Surgeon, Northwest Hospital, Seattle, Washington.
† Associate Professor of Orthopedic Surgery, George Washington University Medical Center, Washington, D.C.
‡ Professor and Chairman, Department of Orthopedic Surgery, George Washington University Medical Center, Washington, D.C.

of the talus, primarily because of loss of a fragment or gross contamination. Six of these had a good result with fibrous ankylosis of the tibiocalcaneal joint. Nevertheless, he recommended arthrodesis as the salvage procedure of choice when primary treatment failed.

In the many studies regarding complications of fractures of the talus, little mention has been made of the severe problem of osteomyelitis. The present study was undertaken to evaluate the results of talectomy for osteomyelitis of the talus.

## MATERIAL AND METHODS

Four patients have been seen since 1968 with osteomyelitis of the talus subsequent to fracture. After the diagnosis of osteomyelitis was established by roentgenographic changes and culture of the drainage, all patients were placed on a program of cast immobilization, systemic antibiotics, and local drainage. One patient underwent partial sequestrectomy of the talus on two occasions without improvement.

All patients underwent talectomy with external rotation and posterior displacement of the foot as described by Whitman.[18] In addition, closed suction irrigation as described by Compere[4] and Clawson[2] was used. The patients were placed in long leg casts with the foot in five to 10 degrees of equinus at the time of surgery. Six weeks postoperatively, a short leg walking cast was applied and partial weight bearing was begun. At three months, external plaster immobilization was discontinued and ambulation on crutches with progressive weight bearing started.

The ages of the patients ranged from 25 to 65 years. The time span from initial injury to talectomy ranged from five to 18 months. The follow-up has been 18 to 65 months with an average of 29 months.

## RESULTS

The goals of surgery were elimination of drainage, a stable, painless tibiocalcaneal fibrous ankylosis, and a satisfactory ambulatory status. These goals were achieved in three of the four patients. Three of the four were rated excellent while one was a failure.

Case 1. A. C., a 39 year old man, sustained a comminuted fracture of the left medial malleolus and a fracture of the body of the talus in a fall from a ladder in 1966. Treatment initially consisted of open reduction and internal fixation of both fractures. In 1969 he still was unable to walk without crutches because of traumatic arthritis of the left ankle and aseptic necrosis of the talus (Fig. 1.). In 1970 he contused the left ankle and developed an open, draining sinus tract which cultured Staphylococcus aureus. When he as first seen in our clinic he was treated by immobilization, local drainage, and systemic antibiotics. He was unimproved after one year and in January 1972 underwent talectomy with closed suction irrigation which was continued for two weeks postoperatively. He remained in a long leg cast for six weeks and then began partial weight bearing in a short leg walking cast. Three months after surgery, plaster immobilization was discontinued and progressive weight bearing was started.

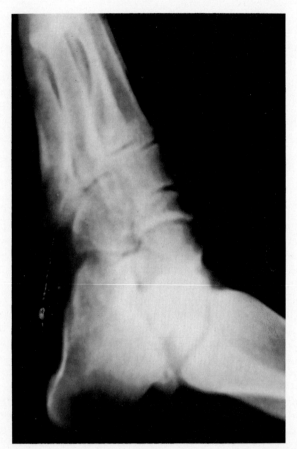

Figure 1.    Thirty-nine year old man with degenerative changes in the ankle joint and avascular changes in the talus. There was a draining sinus from the ankle joint. This roentgenogram was taken four years after injury.

Eighteen months postoperatively he was walking with no external support and had no pain or other limitation. The foot was in excellent alignment and fixed in 10 degrees of equinus (Fig. 2). He was using a 1¼ inch heel lift and a ¾ inch sole lift. There was a fibrous ankylosis of the tibia to the calcaneus. The foot was stable, there had been no drainage from the ankle since surgery, and the patient was satisfied. The result was rated excellent.

CASE 2.    L. T., a 25 year old woman, sustained a severe open, comminuted fracture-dislocation of the right ankle and talus in an automobile accident in February 1971. Ischemia of the foot was present on her arrival in the emergency room. The foot was manually reduced immediately; however, traction had to be maintained to prevent circulatory embarrassment. Under general anesthesia the foot was held in a reduced position and a long leg cast applied and immediately bivalved. Skin necrosis developed postoperatively and failed to heal but was not grafted because of drainage. In May 1971 osteomyelitis of the talus was noted. A draining sinus at the medial malleolus cultured Staphylococcus aureus and Kleb-

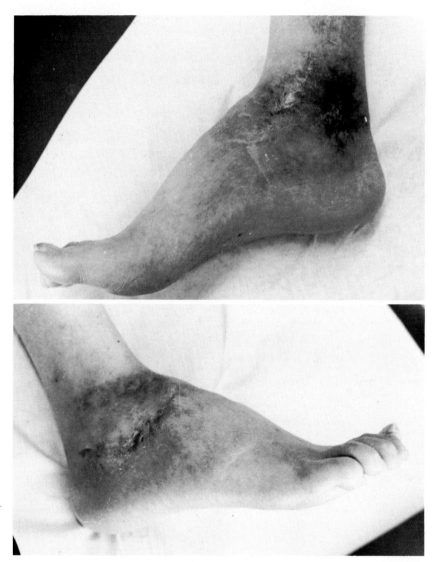

Figure 2.   Same patient seen in Figure 1, 18 months post talectomy. The foot is in excellent alignment and in 10 degrees equinus.

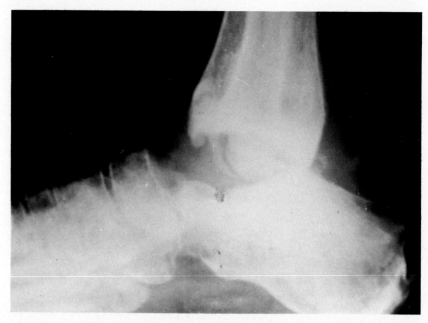

Figure 3.  Relationship of the tibia to the os calcis 18 months post talectomy in a 25 year old woman who had sustained a severe, open, comminuted fracture-dislocation of the right ankle and talus.

siella. She was treated with systemic antibiotics for four months with no improvement. A sinogram was performed which outlined the talus. In October 1971, talectomy (Fig. 3) with closed suction irrigation was performed.

The postoperative treatment was as described in the first case. At 18 months follow-up she could walk and run without external support. The foot was in excellent position and stable in 10 degrees of equinus (Fig. 4). A fibrous ankylosis had been achieved. The patient was using a one-half inch heel lift without complaint. She can now walk five or six miles without fatigue or pain and is active in sports. A rating of excellent was achieved.

CASE 3.   H. S., a 70 year old man, fell from a ladder in 1967 and sustained an open fracture of the ankle with complete dislocation and extrusion of the talus. The talus was removed, cleaned, and replaced within the ankle. Immobilization was achieved by crossed Kirschner wire fixation (Fig. 5A) and application of a long leg cast. When the cast was removed after three months, a draining sinus developed which cultured Staphylococcus aureus. The ankle was drained surgically, and antibiotics were given until the drainage ceased. The draining sinus recurred when the antibiotics were discontinued.

In February 1968, talectomy with closed suction irrigation was performed. Seven weeks postoperatively, the cast was removed and progressive ambulation begun. In May 1973 the foot was in excellent position with zero degrees of equinus (Figs. 5B and 6). A fibrous ankylosis had been achieved. The foot was pain-free and had not drained since surgery. His walking was limited to eight to 10 blocks because of pulmonary insufficiency secondary to a right pneumonec-

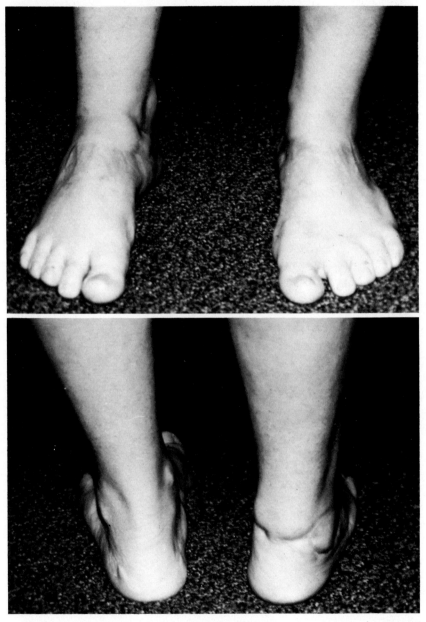

Figure 4.   Same patient seen in Figure 3 with excellent alignment of the foot 18 months postoperatively. The patient is wearing a regular shoe with a ½ inch heel lift. No external support is used.

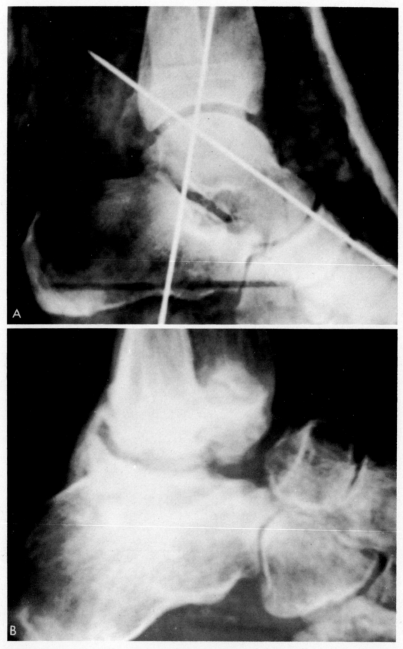

Figure 5.  *A*, A 70 year old man with complete extrusion of the talus. The talus was replaced and immobilized with crossed Kirschner wires. *B*, Sixty-five months post talectomy. The roentgenogram shows the foot placed well posteriorly in relation to the tibia.

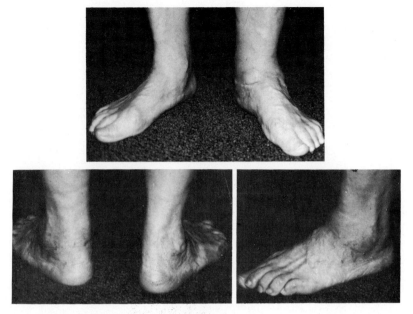

Figure 6.    Same patient seen in Figure 5. Sixty-five months postoperatively the foot is in excellent position with zero degrees equinus.

tomy for bronchogenic carcinoma in 1962. The patient uses a cane only for long walks and has no complaints about his foot. This patient's results were rated excellent.

CASE 4.   J. D., a 29 year old Vietnam veteran, was injured in a land mine explosion in July 1970 and sustained multiple injuries including an open fracture of the right talus. The right ankle wound was debrided initially, and the patient was transferred to medical facilities in the United States. Osteomyelitis was diagnosed soon after his arrival. He underwent sequestrectomy and closed suction irrigation of the right ankle on two occasions (Fig. 7A). The drainage subsided five months after the injury. The patient continued to have pain on weight-bearing with intermittent edema and erythema about the ankle, however drainage did not recur. The patient had a fixed varus deformity of the foot. In January 1972 he underwent talectomy with a valgus osteotomy of the os calcis and tibiocalcaneal arthrodesis with bone grafting and internal fixation. No attempt was made to externally rotate or posteriorly displace the foot; closed suction irrigation was not used.

The arthrodesis failed, and the patient was unable to bear weight on the right foot because of pain and swelling (Fig. 7B). He was placed on antibiotics in August 1972 because of pain, erythema, and swelling of the ankle, as well as an elevated temperature. He was kept on antibiotics for three months with no improvement. In October 1972 a below-knee amputation was performed, and the patient was fitted with a prosthesis. He has had no subsequent problems. This case was classified as a failure.

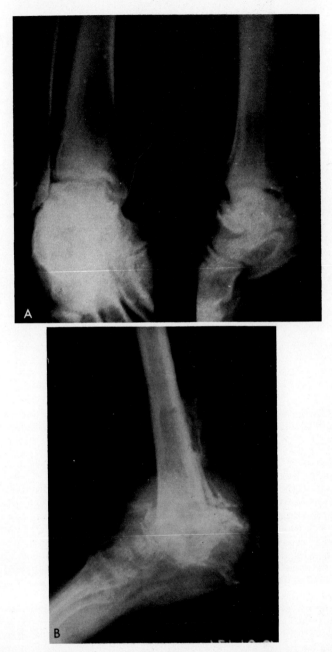

Figure 7. *A*, Osteomyelitis of the talus after open fracture. This patient underwent a sequestrectomy on two occasions. *B*, Seven months postoperatively, talectomy with attempted tibiocalcaneal arthrodesis had failed. The procedure failed to control infection and an amputation below the knee was necessary.

## DISCUSSION

The management of fractures and fracture-dislocations of the talus remains a difficult problem. In rare instances the problem is made more complex by total dislocation of the talus with open fracture. Even in these injuries there have been good results reported for patients treated by debridement and replacement of the talus.[10, 13] Severe infection may be prevented in some patients by excision of the wound and primary skin grafting to obtain coverage. Most recent sutdies advocate arthrodesis of symptomatic joints as a salvage procedure, primarily because of the poor results following talectomy in adults.[3, 6, 11, 12, 14, 15]

Osteomyelitis of the talus is the one condition in which talectomy is indicated.[3, 6, 10, 12] After removal of the talus, if the foot is externally rotated and displaced posteriorly with reference to the tibia, tibiocalcaneal fibrous ankylosis can be obtained with good functional position of the foot. The surgical dissection necessary for arthrodesis is contraindicated in the presence of infection, and bone grafts show poor survival in infected wounds.[9, 19]

The one failure in this study is thought to be a result of technical errors. In this patient an attempt was made to achieve arthrodesis—an end point which is not only unnecessary but undesirable in the presence of infection. In addition, the foot was not properly positioned to allow for a good gait postoperatively. Closed suction irrigation was not used, and the patient eventually required below-knee amputation for relief of pain and control of infection.

The goals of the operation were achieved in three of the four patients. None of these patients was weight bearing on the involved extremity prior to surgery. The most satisfying aspect of the procedure for the patients was their ability to bear full weight without pain and eliminate use of crutches or a cane.

## SUMMARY

In this series excellent results have been achieved by talectomy with external rotation and posterior displacement of the foot. The procedure is not performed to maintain motion at the tibiocalcaneal joint but to achieve painless fibrous ankylosis and eliminate infection. When the procedure is varied, the results may be less than ideal. External support may be required if the foot is not maintained in the recommended position of posterior displacement, external rotation, and between zero and 10 degrees of equinus.

## REFERENCES

1. Cabot, H., and Binney, H.: Fractures of the os calcis and astragalus. Ann. Surg., *45*:51-68, 1907.
2. Clawson, D.K., and Dunn, A. W.: Management of common bacterial infections of bones and joints. J. Bone Joint Surg., *49A*:164, 1967.

3. Coltart, W. D.: Aviator's astragalus J. Bone Joint Surg., 34B:545-566, 1952.

4. Compere, E. L.: Treatment of osteomyelitis and infected wounds by closed irrigation with a detergent antibiotic solution. Acta Orthop. Scand., 32:324-333, 1962.

5. Cooper, A.: Treatise on Dislocations and Fractures of the Joints. Boston, Wells and Lilly, 1818.

6. Dunn, A. R., Jacobs, B., and Campbell, R. D.: Fractures of the talus. J. Trauma, 6:443, 1966.

7. Fabricus, H.: Report Quoted in Opera, Quae Extant Omnia. Beyer Francofurti Ad Moenum, 1646, p. 140.

8. Graham, W. T., and Faulkner, D. M.: Astragalectomy for fractures of the astragalus. Ann. Surg., 89:435, 1939.

9. Judet, R., and Judet, J.: La decortication osteo-periostee: Principle, technique, indications et resultats. Mem. Acad. Chir., 91:463, 1965.

10. Kenwright, J., and Taylor, R. G.: Major injuries of the talus. J. Bone Joint Surg., 52B:36, 1970.

11. McKeever, F. M.: Treatment of complications of fractures and dislocations of the talus. Clin. Orthop., 30:45, 1963.

12. Miller, O. L., and Baker, L. D.: Fracture and fracture-dislocation of the astragalus. South. Med. J., 32:125, 1939.

13. Mindell, E. R., Cisek, E. E., Kartalian, G., et al.: Late results of injuries to the talus. J. Bone Joint Surg., 45A:221, 1963.

14. Pennal, G. F.: Fractures of the talus. Clin. Orthop., 30:53, 1963.

15. Schrock, R. D., Johnson, H. F., and Waters, C. H.: Fractures and fracture-dislocations of the astragalus. J. Bone Joint Surg., 24:560-573, 1942.

16. Stealy, J. H.: Fracture of the astragalus. Surg. Gynecol. Obstet., 8:36-48, 1909.

17. Syme, J.: Contributions to the Pathology and Practice of Surgery. Edition 1. Edinburgh, Sutherland and Knox, 1848, p. 126.

18. Whitman, R.: The operative treatment of paralytic talipes of the calcaneus type. J. Am. Med. Sci., 122:593, 1901.

19. Winter, L.: Management of chronic osteitis and osteomyelitis with a coagulum of autogenous blood, penicillin and thrombin. J. Internat. Chir., 11:510, 1951.

*Chapter 14*

# Experience with Wilson's Oblique Displacement Osteotomy for Hallux Valgus

ARTHUR HOLSTEIN, M.D.*

GWILYM B. LEWIS, M.D.†

The oblique displacement osteotomy for hallux valgus as described by J. N. Wilson[3] had as its primary purpose the treatment of this deformity in adolescence. He felt that the standard procedures used for the correction of this deformity in the middle-aged group were not entirely satisfactory for the younger individuals who are more active and put heavier demands on the operative site. We have found that, in the past, the complaints in both young and the middle-aged patients preoperatively were pain and gross deformity, and the complaints postoperatively were recurrence of deformity and some pain and stiffness in the metatarsophalangeal joint. We therefore undertook to apply this procedure to the young patients, as was advised, and extended it to the older age group, as was "not suggested" by Wilson in 1963.

The method proposed promised to be simple since other osteotomies had been done previously, but they were rendered unnecessarily complicated by their techniques or produced a small distal fragment that required special shaping, and often needed a fixation to render it stable while still not changing the metatarsus primus.[1,2] Also the Wilson procedure listed the following as advantages: a recurrence of only five to 10 degrees to be accepted as normal; no troublesome loss of mobility at the metatarsophalangeal joint of the toe operated; none of the patients showed significant metatarsalgia; union of all osteotomies, but not uniformly so in timing; no pain in the osteotomy site; and finally, a failure rate of only one in 25 operations.

With these as the basic advantages, and in view of limitations of multiple methods we had already used, we undertook the displacement osteotomy as outlined. We have attempted only to alter the age group to

---

* Attending Orthopedic Surgeon, Alta Bates and Herrick Memorial Hospitals, Berkeley, California.
† Attending Orthopedic Surgeon, Alta Bates and Herrick Memorial Hospitals, Berkeley, California.

**Table 1.**  *Materials for Comparison in Two Series of Oblique Displacement Osteotomies for Hallux Valgus*

|                      | WILSON         | HOLSTEIN-LEWIS  |
|----------------------|----------------|-----------------|
| Number of patients   | 24             | 64              |
| Number of procedures | 34             | 98              |
| Age span             | 14 to 49 years | 14 to 77 years  |
| Average age          | 24 years       | 50.5 years      |
| Longest follow-up    | 8 years        | 9 years         |
| Shortest follow-up   | 3 months       | 6 months        |

ascertain whether the method is applicable to the older age group with the same good quality of end results described by Wilson.

## MATERIAL

We have been able to evaluate a series of 98 operations in 64 patients with a follow-up extending back to 1964 (Table 1). The youngest patient was 14 years of age (Fig. 1), the oldest male was 77 years of age (Fig. 2), and the oldest female was 68 years of age. The average age was 50.5 years.

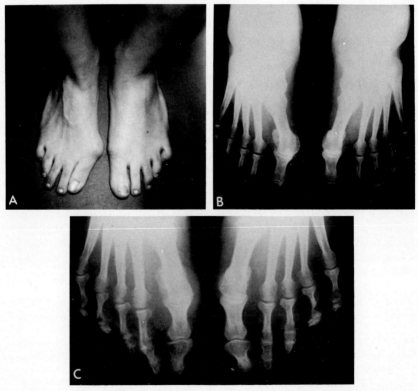

Figure 1.  *A*, Youngest patient, age 14. *B*, Preoperative x-ray film taken of right hallux valgus. *C*, Postoperative position.

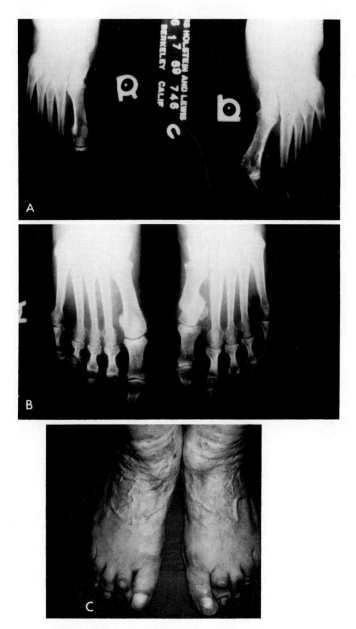

Figure 2. *A*, Oldest patient, age 77. Preoperative hallux valgus of the left foot. *B*, Postoperative position of osteotomy. *C*, Appearance of postoperative position for correction of left hallux valgus.

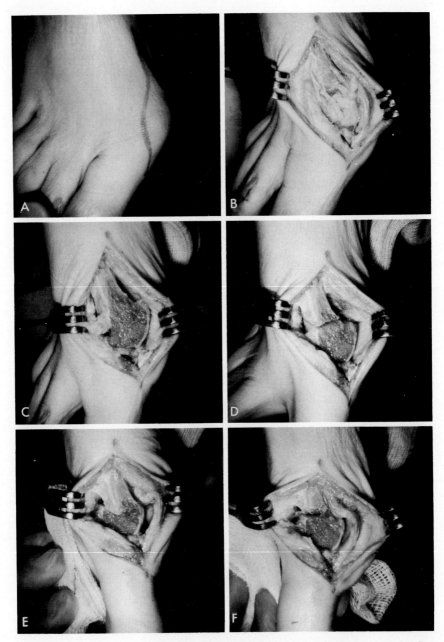

Figure 3. *A*, A curved incision is made on the dorsomedial aspect of the first metatarsophalangeal joint area and the flaps reflected to give visualization of the distal portion of the metatarsal with its exostosis, the capsule, and the base of the phalanx.

*B*, A linear incision is made from the base of the phalanx continuing along the capsule overlying the exostosis and terminating in the periosteum overlying the distal one third of the first metatarsal. The capsule-periosteum was elevated to visualize the exostosis and the medial side of the distal metatarsal shaft, plus elevation of only the periosteum on the plantar and lateral side of the neck of the shaft.

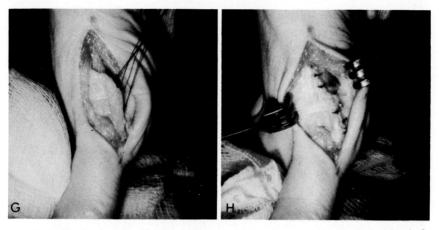

Figure 3. (*Continued*).   *C*, The exostosis on the head is removed in the line of the shaft with an osteotome.

*D*, The osteotomy is made at a 45 degree angle starting distally and medially, and extending laterally and proximally. The distal fragment created in this way should be confined to the distal one third of the metatarsal. We prefer to do this osteotomy with a power saw.

*E*, Displace the distal fragment laterally toward the second metatarsal and rotate the large toe with the distal fragment into wide adduction (medially).

*F*, Rongeur the point of the proximal portion of the shaft so that it is relatively flat with the newly positioned distal fragment.

*G*, Imbricate the capsule with multiple mattress sutures.

*H*, If there is excessive capsular tissue remaining, this can be removed, or the free edge overlapped and sutured down. This produces a firm medial ligament and helps prevent displacement of the distal fragment. Immobilization is then carried out in a below-knee plaster with phalanx held in position of correction by a plaster wedge.

In addition to the pain factor and deformity of the hallux valgus common to both series, the older age group had 36 hammer toe deformities, 12 overlapping of the second phalanx on the first, four subluxations or frank dislocations of the metatarsophalangeal joints—which required correction at the same time that the oblique osteotomies were carried out.

## SURGICAL PROCEDURE

The operative procedure is described in detail and illustrated in Figure 3, *A* to *H*. Modifications in the original procedure have been kept at a minimum. These modifications include the handling and imbrication of the capsule as described rather than the creation of a flap that is based distally, the use of the power saw blade for the osteotomy rather than the osteotome, and the trimming of the point on the proximal osteotomy fragment. The aftercare immobilization was eight weeks in duration. We modified this by not removing the wedge between the first and second toes until the fourth to sixth weeks in order to protect the osteotomy site. We did the skin closure with plain catgut interrupted sutures to avoid the need for disturbing the immobilization if it was comfortable. After the removal of the plaster, the foot was fitted with a shoe that had a neutral medial last.

## RESULTS

The interval of time from treatment of the first patient to the present is nine years, as compared with eight years in Wilson's series. The evaluation of patients was carried out using the same categories (Table 2).

RECURRENCE OF DEFORMITY. The cosmetic end result has been uniformly good. We have a marked recurrence of the deformity in one patient and a partial recurrence of more than half of the correction in three patients.

MOBILITY OF THE METATARSOPHALANGEAL JOINT. There has been a maintenance of mobility in all patients except one, and this patient was subsequently treated by Keller procedure. This patient had undergone prior surgery that had failed. In this series, there were 10 patients who had prior bunion surgery.

METATARSALGIA. Here there was a significant increase in complaints as compared with the original presentation. A total of 17 patients reported metatarsalgia, nine of whom requested treatment consisting of

**Table 2.** *Summary of Results Based on Number of Procedures*

|  | WILSON | HOLSTEIN-LEWIS |
| --- | --- | --- |
| Recurrence of deformity | | |
|   (5 to 10° valgus normal) | 34 procedures | 98 procedures |
|     Complete | 1 | 1 |
|     Partial | 2 | 3 |
| Limited mobility of metatarso- | | |
|   phalangeal joint | 0 | 1 |
| Metatarsalgia—total | 7 | 17 |
|   Temporary needing no treatment | 6 | 8 |
|   Persistent | 1 | 9 |
|     Secondary surgery | 0 | 1 |
|     Acquired fracture, second | | |
|       metatarsal | 0 | 1 |
| Rate of union | | |
|   Clinical union at 8 weeks | All | All |
|   Nonunion | 0 | 0 |
|   Malunion | 1 | 2 |
| Pain in osteotomy site or first metatarso- | | |
|   phalangeal joint* | 1 | 2 |
| Infection | 0 | 1 |

* Same as malunion.

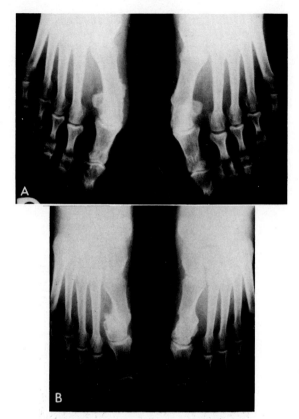

Figure 4. *A*, X-ray film showing recurrence of bilateral hallux valgus in prior Silver procedures. *B*, X-ray film showing realignment of hallux valgus recurrence by oblique displacement osteotomy.

the use of a pad in the shoe or a metatarsal bar; one of these patients subsequently underwent a resection of the head of the second metatarsal, and one patient developed a March fracture of the second metatarsal. Only two patients in this group with metatarsalgia were under 49 years of age.

RATE OF UNION. None showed gross bony union on x-ray films taken prior to eight weeks after surgery. None failed to unite. Three months was the average time of demonstrable bony union.

PAIN IN OSTEOTOMY-BUNIONECTOMY AREA. Six patients reported some pain in the first metatarsal area at some time during follow-up. In only two (same patients) was it sufficiently persistent to require treatment, which consisted of dorsal exostectomy.

INFECTION. One patient developed postoperative infection—*Staphylococcus aureus*—that occurred seven weeks postoperatively and was quiescent in three weeks.

## CONCLUSION

We have found that the oblique displacement osteotomy has resulted in uniformly good correction of the pain and deformity resulting from hallux valgus. This is especially true where metatarsus adductus is a primary factor (Fig. 5). We have found that the method originally designed for the adolescent and the young adult can be safely and successfully extended to the middle-aged patient. In doing so, the factor of metatarsalgia, either in the second and third areas or in the osteotomized component, has been introduced into the end result with greater frequency in the older age group. We are making no effort in this report to indicate whether this situation existed preoperatively. There were no nonunions however an infection developed in one patient. The cosmet-

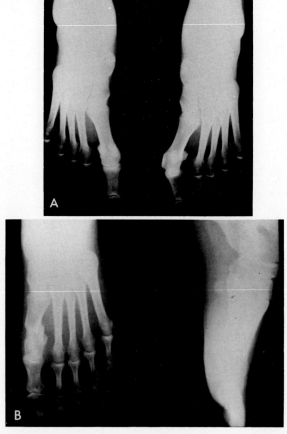

Figure 5. *A*, X-ray film showing preoperative hallux valgus with the primary component being metatarsus adductus. *B*, X-ray film showing postoperative realignment by oblique displaced osteotomy.

ic appearance has been uniformly better than we have been able to obtain by the other methods we have used, especially when the deformity is marked. The recurrence rate for the deformity has been less frequent with the oblique displacement osteotomy. If one is hesitant to use the oblique displacement osteotomy as an initial procedure, the method is also effective for correction of recurrence from other procedures (Fig. 4).

## REFERENCES

1. Carr, C. R., and Boyd, B. M.: Correctional osteotomy for metatarsus primus varus and hallux valgus. J. Bone Joint Surg., *48A*:1649. 1966.

2. Mitchell, C. L., Fleming, J. L., Allen, R., et al.: Osteotomy and bunionectomy for hallux valgus. J. Bone Joint Surg., *40A*:141, 1958.

3. Wilson, J. N.: Oblique displacement osteotomy for hallux valgus. J. Bone Joint Surg., *45B*:552, 1963.

*Chapter 15*

# Hallux Valgus—Surgical Correction by Three-in-One Technique

RALPH T. LIDGE, M.D.*

The choice of surgical correction procedures for hallux valgus is bewildering. The textbooks of Kelikian,[10] Giannestras,[6] and DuVries,[5] and others with their respective author index and article reference serve to confirm this feeling. The author of this paper has employed many techniques over the years, some old and some new, but the overall end result in many instances has not been as favorable as anticipated. During the last five years a plan or method has been evolved that to date has given more satisfactory results. The technique is a blending of the old and the new, aided by power instrumentation now available. This method appears to be adaptable to all age groups. This chapter presents a procedure, parts of which may be used as a simple or combined method, for the treatment of hallux valgus in all age groups.

## DEFINITION

According to Kelikian,[10] hallux valgus is present when the angle at the metatarsophalangeal joint exceeds an inclination of 8 to 10 degrees. Medial deviation of the first metatarsal is combined with lateral flexion of the big toe. The deformity is considered as simple with the above angulation when it is not associated with axial rotation of the big toe. The angle between the first and second metatarsal and the metatarsus varus primus angle should not be greater than 8 to 9 degrees in the majority of feet according to Hardy and Clapham,[8] and no greater than 10 degrees according to Durman.[4]

In measuring the angle of hallux valgus, the angle created by the intersection of a line representing the long axis of the first metatarsal and of the proximal phalanx is studied. For the metatarsus intermetatarsal

---

* Clinical Assistant Professor of Orthopedic Surgery, The Abraham Lincoln School of Medicine, University of Illinois Medical Center, Chicago; Attending Staff, Lutheran General Hospital, Park Ridge, Illinois and Northwest Community Hospital, Arlington Heights, Illinois.

angle, or the degree of metatarsus varus primus, an angle created by the two lines, each running in the longitudinal axis of their respective metatarsal, is utilized.

## ETIOLOGY

In 1871 Heuter[9] first described the deformity of hallux valgus as an abduction contracture, that is, a deviation of the big toe laterally from the median plane of the body. DuVries[5] believed that variation in the contour of the base of the first metatarsal was an important factor. McElvenny[12] and Truslow[15] considered heredity to be a strong underlying cause. Giannestras[6] contends that there is a basic structural defect of the foot which predisposes to the development of this deformity. Ill-fitting shoes may accentuate the situation and contribute to the development of the bunion.

The underlying cause may very well be hereditary but the ultimate deformity is the result of the combined forces exerted at the metatarsophalangeal joint, and the metatarsotarsal joint together with the intrinsic shape of the two respective joint areas.

## ANATOMY AND PATHOMECHANICS

According to Spalteholz,[14] the oblique head of the adductor hallucis is fused medially with lateral belly of the flexor hallucis brevis, and this forms a conjoined tendon. The transverse belly of the adductor hallucis, together with the conjoined tendon, insert into the lateral sesmoid and are prolonged into the base of the first phalanx of the great toe, the purpose of which is to plantar flex and laterally deviate the big toe. The medial belly of the flexor hallucis brevis attaches to the base of the proximal phalanx on its medial side. En route, its tendon contains the tibial sesmoid and it acts as a plantar flexor. The abductor hallucis also connects to the medial sesmoid as well as to the base of the proximal phalanx on the medial side and deviates the big toe medially and plantarly. The extensor hallucis longus often is connected by thin bands to the proximal phalanx of the big toe and inserts into the base of the second toe. It dorsiflexes as well as pronates and abducts the foot and also extends the big toe dorsally. The extensor hallucis brevis passing obliquely across the dorsum of the foot is inserted into the dorsal surface of the base of the proximal phalanx, acting as a dorsiflexor. The flexor hallucis longus flexes the foot plantarly and supinates and adducts as well, and attaches to the proximal part of the second phalanx.

The author has noted that, associated with the overall increased strength of the adductor hallucis over the abductor hallucis, there also develops a bony overgrowth or increase in length of the tibial cortex of the proximal phalanx of the big toe as compared with the fibular side. The medial capsular structures become overstretched, the lateral become contracted. The long toe extensor then acts more as a lateral deviator of the big toe together with extending it and shows a lateral shift. In many instances the long toe extensor becomes shortened; it assists in further pronation of the big toe together with the flexor hallucis.

DuVries[5] describes the shift of the fibular sesmoid as being lateral so that it becomes the hub of the deformity, being moved by the combined pull of the heads of the adductor hallucis. Thus concomitant soft tissue changes occur manifested by contracture of the fibular joint capsule and overstretching of the tibial portion of the metatarsophalangeal joint capsule.

## TECHNIQUE

The surgical procedure effected under tourniquet control can be divided into three parts. The first part is universally employed and is combined with the second or third portions, or both.

The first aspect—a modification of the Silver[13] procedure—is carried out essentially as follows. A longitudinally curved incision is made over the dorsal medial aspect of the metatarsophalangeal joint (Fig. 1). The incision is more medial than dorsal in order to avoid trauma to the cutaneous sensory branch of the superficial peroneal nerve. A Y-shaped incision is then made through the medial joint capsule leaving the capsule attached to the proximal phalanx with a long portion of the Y extending along the distal metatarsal. The metatarsophalangeal joint is exposed and the medial prominence of the head of the metatarsal is resectioned (Fig. 2). Traction is maintained on the big toe and section is carried out on the lateral capsule together with the lateral collateral ligament and adductor hallucis tendon. The final procedure in the modified Silver technique is performed following the osteotomy of either the metatarsal or proximal phalanx, or both. The triangular capsular complex is advanced proximally and attached to the soft tissue along the medial side of the metatarsal with imbrication of the residual dorsal and plantar flaps in the local area with the abductor hallucis portion being included in the plantar flap.

The second phase of the technique involves an osteotomy of the proximal metatarsal if so indicated. This reduces the angle between the first and second metatarsals. As pointed out by Kelikian,[10] this procedure was first suggested by Loison[11] in 1901, namely, a cuneiform osteotomy of the proximal metatarsal distal to the insertion of the long peroneal tendon. Balacesu[2] was the first to perform the surgery in 1903. A longitudinal incision is made over the proximal first metatarsal lateral to the long extensor tendon. Through this incision, a lateral closing wedge osteotomy of the proximal part of the first metatarsal is carried out. This is performed with the aid of an oscillating power saw. The medial cortex is broken by a greenstick-like fracture and fixation is secured by one, or possibly two, transfixion Kirschner wires .062 inch in diameter. The medial portion of the wire should protrude from the medial cortex sufficiently to facilitate its removal at a later date.

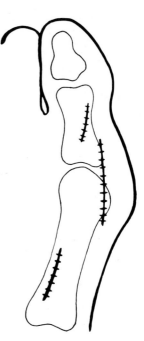

Figure 1. Surgical approach for each procedure for correction of hallux valgus. The distal two incisions may be connected if desired.

The third phase is that of osteotomy of the base of the proximal phalanx (Fig. 3). Akin[1] in 1925 and Giannestras[7] in 1972 recommended this method as a primary procedure for the age group of 40 to 65. However the author believes the technique is useful in all age groups where surgical correction is indicated. An incision is made over the proximal part of the proximal phalanx just medial to the long toe extensor. Again the bone is exposed in a subperiosteal manner and a medial closing wedge osteotomy performed with the aid of the power saw. The lateral cortex is then broken by manual manipulation, and fixation is secured by an intramedullary Kirschner wire .062 inch in diameter extending through the distal phalanx into the two parts of the proximal phalanx, through the metatarsophalangeal joint, maintaining the big toe in the correct position. The Kirschner wire through the metatarsophalangeal joint gives a better overall end result since the metatarsophalangeal joint is fixed for a short period of time and the soft tissue may then heal about the metatarsophalangeal joint in the corrected position; it also reduces the amount of postoperative discomfort. The pin is bent at right angles just beyond its point of protrusion at the tip of the toe and cut so as to be prominent for a few millimeters. The attention is directed again, as indicated above, to the first incision over the dorsal medial aspect of the metatarsophalangeal joint, and at this time the capsular flap is advanced proximally together with suture to the local soft tissue and imbrication of the dorsal and plantar flaps, as described above.

Only if the first metatarsal is osteotomized is the foot placed in a cast with first a short leg posterior plaster splint for five to seven days and

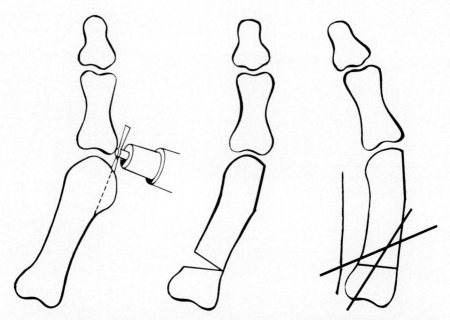

Figure 2. The use of a light-weight oscillating power saw is of inestimable value. The lateral closing wedge osteotomy is transfixed preferably by two crossed heavy Kirschner wires, one wire transfixing the osteotomy site, the other engaging the adjacent metatarsal. The wedge of bone removed is inserted laterally as a graft at the osteotomy location.

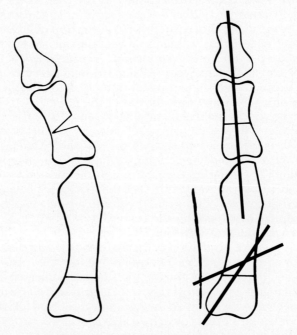

Figure 3. The intramedullary Kirschner wire should cross the metatarsal phalangeal joint to maintain alignment of the big toe.

thereafter with a circular cast with weight bearing permitted after three weeks. The pin is removed from the big toe in four weeks. The cast is taken off in six weeks and the metatarsal pins extracted at that time.

The expected average duration of follow-up for outpatient visits following discharge from the hospital is about two to three months, depending upon the number of procedures employed.

In patients in whom a modified Silver procedure[13] or a proximal phalanx osteotomy or both have been carried out, care should be taken to employ sufficient wrapping in a proper manner to facilitate maintenance of good position of the metatarsophalangeal joint. The patient may utilize crutches and bear weight as desired, with weight bearing directed toward the heel of the foot.

## CLINICAL EXPERIENCE

A total of 57 consecutive patients, 53 women and four men, were studied and served as the basis of clinical studies, encompassing a total of 92 feet with hallux valgus, 22 unilateral and 35 bilateral.

The patients have been divided into three age groups: juvenile (ages 12 to 20), three unilateral and 18 bilateral, or a total of 39 feet; adult (ages 21 to 55), 10 unilateral and nine bilateral, or a total of 28 feet; and senior group (56 to 70 years of age), nine unilateral and eight bilateral, or a total of 25 feet.

Figure 4 illustrates the age distribution and shows eight patients aged 12 to 15, and 13 patients aged 16 to 20. There is then a marked drop-off in the early phase of the adult group, namely, one patient aged 21 to 25, and two for each of the following age groups—26 to 30, 31 to

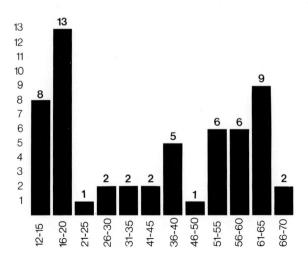

Figure 4.   Number of patients in each age group.

35, and 36 to 40—with five patients in the 41 to 45 group, and then a drop-off to one in the 46 to 50 group, and a sudden rise to six in the age group 51 to 55. The senior age group continues with the increased amount of patients, six in age group 56 to 60, nine in age group 61 to 65, and a drop-off of two in age group 66 to 70. Generally one notes the rather high incidence in the juvenile group with low incidence in the early adult group, a peaking in the 41 to 45 group, and then a drop-off and sudden rise in the 51 to 55 group, continuing with the senior group until a decrease is noted in the age group 66 to 70.

In the juvenile group, metatarsal osteotomy was performed in 16 patients, proximal phalanx osteotomy in two patients, and combined metatarsal and proximal phalanx osteotomy in 21 patients. In the adult group, metatarsal osteotomy was performed in three patients, proximal phalanx osteotomy in nine patients, and combined metatarsal and proximal phalanx osteotomy in 16 patients. In the senior group, metatarsal osteotomy was performed in only one patient, proximal phalanx osteotomy in 10 patients, and combined metatarsal proximal phalanx osteotomy in 14 patients.

Therefore metatarsal osteotomy was performed on 20 feet, proximal phalanx osteotomy on 21 feet, and combined metatarsal and proximal phalanx osteotomy on 51 feet; therefore, metatarsal osteotomies were performed on 71 feet and proximal phalanx osteotomies on 72 feet.

## RESULTS

The length of follow-up in 57 patients was as follow: less than one year, 11; one to two years, 25; three to four years, eight; and four to five years, five.

In the juvenile age group (Fig. 5), in 21 patients 31 feet were measured. The hallux valgus angle preoperatively showed a range of 12 to 45 degrees, postoperatively 0 to 30 degrees; the mode preoperatively was 20, postoperatively 0; the median preoperatively was 25, postoperatively 9. The metatarsus varus primus angle preoperative range was 10 to 20 degrees, postoperative 0 to 10 degrees; the mode preoperatively was 10, postoperatively 0; the median preoperatively was 12, postoperatively 4.

In the adult age group (Figs. 6 and 7) a total number of 19 feet were measured. The hallux valgus range angle preoperatively was 10 to 40 degrees, postoperatively 0 to 20 degrees; the mode preoperatively was 25 and 30, postoperatively 10; the median preoperatively was 26, postoperatively 8. The metatarsus varus primus angle in this group showed a preoperative range of 4 to 16 degrees, postoperatively 0 to 12 degrees; the mode preoperatively was 12, and postoperatively 10; the median preoperatively was 11, postoperatively 6.

In the senior age group (Figs. 8 to 10) a total of 16 feet were measured. The hallux valgus angle in the senior age group preoperatively ranged from 20 to 45 degrees, postoperatively 10 to 20 degrees; the mode preoperatively was 30, postoperatively 10; the median preoperatively was 33, and postoperatively 12. The metatarsus varus primus angle preoperatively ranged from 10 to 26 degrees, postoperatively 0 to 15 degrees; the mode preoperatively was 15, postoperatively 10; the median preoperatively was 16, postoperatively 10 (Tables 1 to 5).

The results were not only analyzed from the anatomical standpoint by angular measurements, but also from a subjective point of view. Patients were circularized as well as examined.

The method of grading (Table 6) regarding subjective and objective function was taken largely from Bonney and Macnab.[3] Please refer to Tables 7 and 8 regarding symptoms and motion of the big toe before and after surgery.

It is interesting to note that of 24 replies regarding overall feeling as far as the big toe was concerned, 19 (79.16 per cent) were satisfied with the results, three (12.50 per cent) felt there was some improvement but were not entirely satisfied, and two (8.34 per cent) were dissatisfied. Again of the 24 who responded, 22 (91.66 per cent) would recommend the operation to someone else with the same problem, and two (8.34 per cent) gave a negative reply.

## COMPLICATIONS

There was incomplete correction at the site of proximal phalanx osteotomy in only one patient, and there were no instances of delayed or nonunion.

Approximately 20 per cent of the patients showed mild swelling after three months of follow-up care; these were usually the patients in whom the combined three-in-one technique had been used.

In 5 per cent of the patients pin migration occurred, that is, further seating of the pin in the foot. It is now felt that this could have been prevented if the pin had been allowed to project beyond the edges of the skin. In 2 per cent of the patients fracture of the pin occurred, the protruding part of the pin beyond the skin being easily removed, the remaining portion of the pin still being within the confines of the foot.

Joint stiffness after surgery that was greater than that experienced preoperatively was present in about 8 per cent of the patients. One patient sustained a fall after the proximal phalanx had healed. There was only minimal displacement at the fracture site and the bone healed uneventfully following simple immobilization in a shoe with a cutout for the big toe.

## SUMMARY

A technique is presented utilizing three methods of correction, the first of which is uniformly employed, and the second and/or third as indicated.

In the juvenile group, if the intermetatarsal angle is 10 degrees or greater, consideration is given to a proximal lateral closing wedge os-

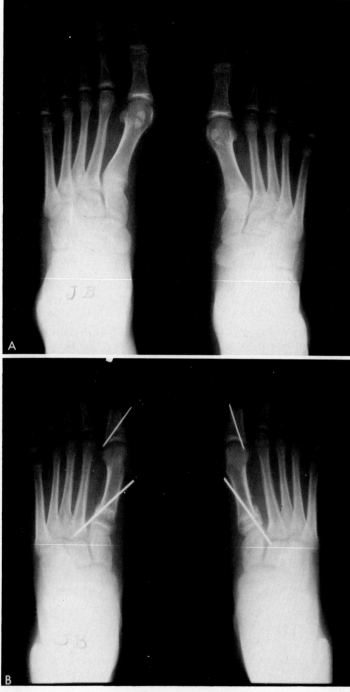

Figure 5. *A*, Juvenile hallux valgus symptomatic in a girl 13½ years of age. *B*, Following removal of casts, x-ray films showed satisfactory healing at osteotomy sites. Note oblique Kirschner wire fixation in both bones.

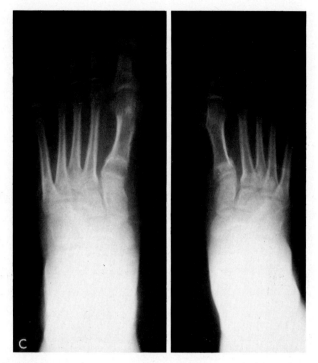

Figure 5 *(Continued)*. *C*, Follow-up x-ray films show that the feet are asymptomatic.

teotomy of the first metatarsal. If the hallux valgus angle exceeds 10 degrees, a medial closing wedge osteotomy of the proximal phalanx is preferred.

In the adult age group, a metatarsal varus primus angle 15 degrees or greater is considered to be an indication for osteotomy of the first metatarsal and, likewise, an angle of 15 degrees or greater for osteotomy of the proximal phalanx.

In the senior age group, a metatarsal varus primus angle of 15 degrees or more is considered to be an indication for metatarsal osteotomy, and a hallux valgus angle of 20 degrees or more for osteotomy of the proximal phalanx.

The modified Silver procedure, when carried out as the sole procedure, is limited to those patients in whom the hallux valgus and the intermetatarsal angles do not exceed the measurements indicated.

The advantages of this procedure are its simplicity and adaptability to various age groups. The results can be expected to be favorable in the majority of patients, the recurrence rate is held to a minimum, the cartilaginous surface of the proximal phalanx and of the head of the metatarsal per se, the metatarsophalangeal joint, is not violated, and reasonably good motion can be expected.

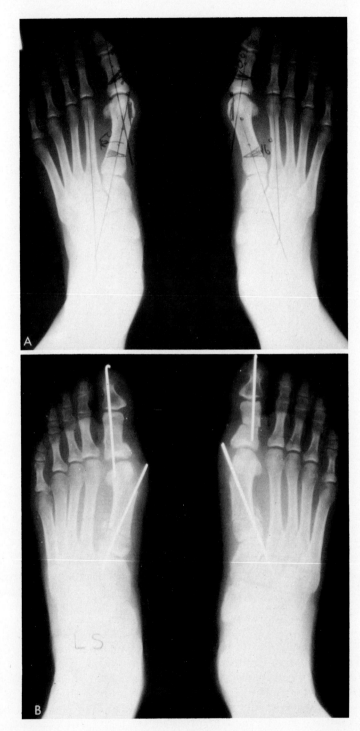

Figure 6.   *(See legend on the opposite page.)*

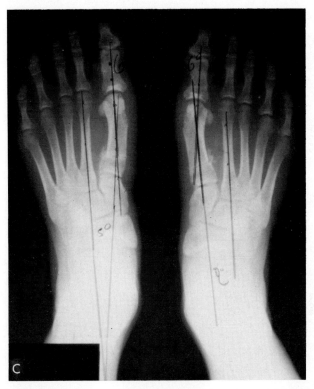

Figure 6.   *A*, A 21 year old woman with bilateral hallux valgus. Right hallux valgus angle is 25 degrees; the left is 30 degrees. The right intermetatarsal angle is 15 degrees; the left is 16 degrees. *B*, This postsurgical x-ray film was taken after removal of casts. *C*, Postsurgical x-ray film. Right and left hallux valgus angle is 6 degrees. The right intermetatarsal angle is 2 degrees; the left is 5 degrees.

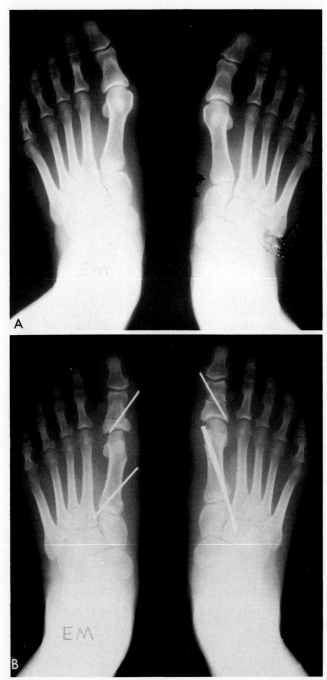

Figure 7.  *A*, A 35 year old woman with symptomatic bilateral hallux valgus. Note increase in length of medial cortex compared with lateral cortex of proximal phalanx of big toe. *B*, Postsurgical x-ray film. Plaster casts are removed, ready for pin extraction.

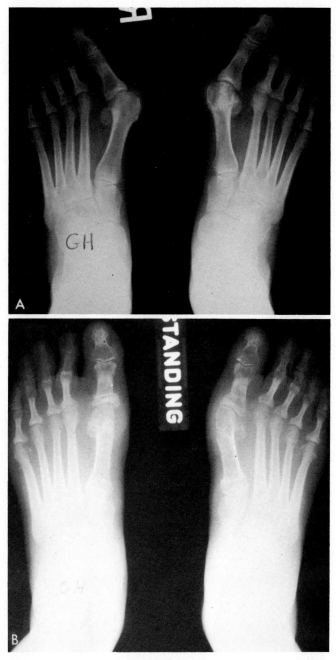

Figure 8. *A*, A 51 year old woman with hallux valgus complicated by drift and pronation deformity of the big toe, especially on right. *B*, This postsurgical x-ray film was taken after the three-in-one technique was performed. Note residual hallux valgus angulation on the right side, thought to result from inadequate release of lateral capsule, including collateral as well as a section of adductor hallucis, and inadequate proximal advancement of medial capsule.

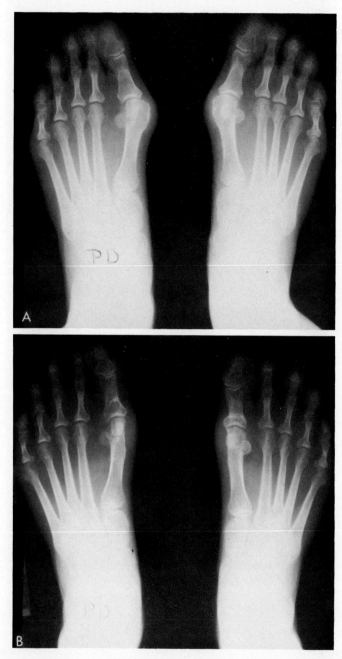

Figure 9. *A*, A 54 year old woman with painful hallux valgus. Note drift deformity of the big toe. *B*, This x-ray film was taken nine months after modified Silver bunionplasty was performed together with medial closing wedge osteotomy of proximal phalanx.

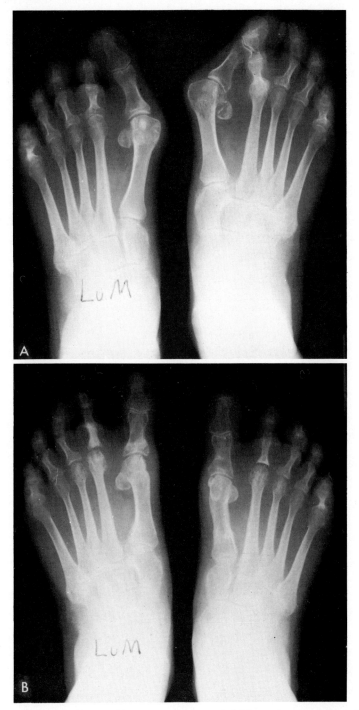

Figure 10.  *A*, A 59 year old woman with very painful feet, who claimed that she was
"unable to obtain decent looking shoes." *B*, This postsurgical x-ray film was taken one year
later. The patient did not have pain at this time.

**Table 1.** *Measurement of Hallux Valgus Angle and Metatarsus Varus Primus Angle in 31 Feet of 21 Patients in the Juvenile Age Group (Ages 12 to 20)*

HALLUX VALGUS ANGLE

| Preoperative | | Postoperative | |
|---|---|---|---|
| Degrees | Number | Degrees | Number |
| 12 | 1 | 0 | 7 |
| 15 | 1 | 2 | 2 |
| 18 | 1 | 5 | 3 |
| 20 | 13 | 6 | 3 |
| 25 | 5 | 8 | 2 |
| 30 | 7 | 10 | 5 |
| 35 | 1 | 12 | 1 |
| 40 | 1 | 15 | 3 |
| 45 | 1 | 20 | 4 |
| | | 30 | 1 |

METATARSUS VARUS PRIMUS ANGLE

| | | | |
|---|---|---|---|
| 10 | 15 | 0 | 15 |
| 12 | 4 | 2 | 1 |
| 14 | 1 | 3 | 1 |
| 15 | 9 | 4 | 2 |
| 18 | 1 | 6 | 3 |
| 20 | 1 | 8 | 4 |
| | | 10 | 5 |

**Table 2.**  *Measurement of Hallux Valgus Angle and Metatarsus*
*Varus Primus Angle in 19 Feet of 19 Patients*
*in the Adult Age Group (Ages 21 to 55)*

HALLUX VALGUS ANGLE

| Preoperative | | Postoperative | |
|---|---|---|---|
| Degrees | Number | Degrees | Number |
| 18 | 1 | 0 | 2 |
| 20 | 4 | 5 | 2 |
| 22 | 1 | 6 | 5 |
| 25 | 5 | 8 | 1 |
| 28 | 1 | 10 | 6 |
| 30 | 5 | 12 | 1 |
| 40 | 2 | 15 | 1 |
|  |  | 20 | 1 |

METATARSUS VARUS PRIMUS ANGLE

| | | | |
|---|---|---|---|
| 4 | 1 | 0 | 3 |
| 6 | 1 | 2 | 1 |
| 10 | 3 | 4 | 2 |
| 12 | 9 | 5 | 2 |
| 14 | 1 | 6 | 3 |
| 15 | 2 | 8 | 1 |
| 16 | 1 | 10 | 5 |
| 18 | 1 | 12 | 1 |
|  |  | 14 | 1 |

**Table 3.**  *Measurement of Hallux Valgus Angle and Metatarsus*
*Varus Primus Angle in 16 Feet in 17 Patients in the*
*Senior Age Group (Ages 56 to 70)*

HALLUX VALGUS ANGLE

| Preoperative | | Postoperative | |
|---|---|---|---|
| Degrees | Number | Degrees | Number |
| 20 | 2 | 10 | 9 |
| 25 | 2 | 12 | 3 |
| 30 | 7 | 15 | 2 |
| 40 | 4 | 16 | 1 |
| 45 | 1 | 20 | 1 |

METATARSUS VARUS PRIMUS ANGLE

| | | | |
|---|---|---|---|
| 10 | 1 | 0 | 1 |
| 14 | 1 | 4 | 1 |
| 15 | 6 | 6 | 1 |
| 16 | 3 | 8 | 2 |
| 18 | 2 | 10 | 5 |
| 20 | 2 | 12 | 3 |
| 26 | 1 | 15 | 3 |

**Table 4.** *Comparison of Results in the Juvenile Age Group*

| AGE | METATARSUS VARUS PRIMUS ANGLE* | | HALLUX VALGUS ANGLE* | | METATARSAL OSTEOTOMY | PROXIMAL PHALANX OSTEOTOMY |
|---|---|---|---|---|---|---|
| | Right | Left | Right | Left | | |
| 15 | $\frac{15}{8}$ | — | $\frac{20}{8}$ | — | + | + |
| 13 | $\frac{10}{10}$ | $\frac{10}{0}$ | $\frac{20}{2}$ | $\frac{20}{6}$ | + | + |
| 14 | $\frac{12}{0}$ | $\frac{10}{0}$ | $\frac{35}{15}$ | $\frac{20}{10}$ | + | + |
| 12 | $\frac{12}{3}$ | $\frac{15}{0}$ | $\frac{25}{0}$ | $\frac{30}{10}$ | + | + |
| 17 | $\frac{15}{10}$ | $\frac{15}{6}$ | $\frac{20}{10}$ | $\frac{15}{5}$ | + | — |
| 16 | $\frac{15}{10}$ | $\frac{15}{8}$ | $\frac{40}{20}$ | $\frac{45}{15}$ | + | + |
| 17 | $\frac{10}{0}$ | — | $\frac{18}{6}$ | — | + | + |
| 14 | $\frac{15}{6}$ | $\frac{12}{6}$ | $\frac{30}{20}$ | $\frac{30}{10}$ | + | — |
| 16 | $\frac{10}{8}$ | $\frac{10}{10}$ | $\frac{20}{15}$ | $\frac{25}{30}$ | + | — |
| 17 | $\frac{10}{0}$ | $\frac{10}{0}$ | $\frac{20}{0}$ | $\frac{30}{0}$ | + | — |
| 16 | $\frac{14}{0}$ | — | $\frac{20}{5}$ | — | + | + |
| 16 | $\frac{20}{0}$ | $\frac{18}{4}$ | $\frac{25}{0}$ | $\frac{25}{6}$ | + | + |
| 16 | $\frac{10}{0}$ | $\frac{15}{0}$ | $\frac{25}{2}$ | $\frac{30}{0}$ | + | + |
| 19 | $\frac{14}{0}$ | $\frac{10}{0}$ | $\frac{20}{0}$ | $\frac{20}{0}$ | + | — |
| 18 | $\frac{10}{0}$ | $\frac{10}{0}$ | $\frac{20}{5}$ | $\frac{12}{10}$ | + | + |
| 14 | $\frac{10}{4}$ | $\frac{10}{10}$ | $\frac{30}{20}$ | $\frac{20}{20}$ | + | + |
| 15 | $\frac{12}{8}$ | $\frac{15}{0}$ | $\frac{20}{12}$ | $\frac{30}{8}$ | + | — |

* Preoperative

Postoperative

**Table 5.** *Comparison of Results in the Adult (Ages 21 to 55) and Senior (Ages 56 to 70) Age Groups*

| AGE | METATARSUS VARUS PRIMUS ANGLE* | | HALLUX VALGUS ANGLE* | | METATARSAL OSTEOTOMY | PROXIMAL PHALANX OSTEOTOMY |
|---|---|---|---|---|---|---|
| | Right | Left | Right | Left | | |
| 44 | — | $\frac{10}{10}$ | — | $\frac{22}{12}$ | — | + |
| 51 | $\frac{12}{10}$ | $\frac{10}{10}$ | $\frac{28}{10}$ | $\frac{20}{8}$ | — | + |
| 40 | — | $\frac{15}{5}$ | — | $\frac{30}{6}$ | + | + |
| 54 | $\frac{12}{12}$ | $\frac{12}{10}$ | $\frac{25}{5}$ | $\frac{30}{10}$ | — | + |
| 43 | $\frac{18}{0}$ | — | $\frac{40}{6}$ | — | + | + |
| 51 | $\frac{10}{8}$ | $\frac{12}{10}$ | $\frac{30}{6}$ | $\frac{40}{20}$ | + | + |
| 29 | $\frac{12}{0}$ | — | $\frac{18}{0}$ | — | + | + |
| 51 | $\frac{6}{4}$ | $\frac{4}{4}$ | $\frac{20}{10}$ | $\frac{20}{10}$ | — | + |
| 35 | $\frac{12}{6}$ | $\frac{12}{0}$ | $\frac{20}{5}$ | $\frac{25}{0}$ | + | + |
| 27 | $\frac{12}{6}$ | $\frac{12}{6}$ | $\frac{25}{10}$ | $\frac{25}{10}$ | — | + |
| 21 | $\frac{15}{5}$ | $\frac{16}{2}$ | $\frac{25}{6}$ | $\frac{30}{6}$ | + | + |
| 55 | $\frac{14}{14}$ | | $\frac{30}{15}$ | | — | + |
| **SENIOR AGE GROUP** | | | | | | |
| 59 | $\frac{20}{8}$ | $\frac{26}{10}$ | $\frac{40}{10}$ | $\frac{30}{10}$ | + | + |
| 67 | $\frac{14}{10}$ | $\frac{18}{14}$ | $\frac{30}{16}$ | $\frac{30}{15}$ | — | + |
| 61 | — | $\frac{15}{15}$ | — | $\frac{20}{10}$ | — | + |
| 59 | $\frac{18}{6}$ | — | $\frac{25}{10}$ | — | + | + |
| 61 | $\frac{15}{4}$ | — | $\frac{40}{10}$ | — | + | + |
| 65 | — | $\frac{20}{8}$ | — | $\frac{40}{10}$ | + | + |
| 60 | $\frac{15}{15}$ | $\frac{15}{15}$ | $\frac{30}{10}$ | $\frac{25}{12}$ | — | + |
| 61 | — | $\frac{10}{10}$ | — | $\frac{30}{12}$ | — | + |
| 56 | — | $\frac{16}{0}$ | — | $\frac{40}{10}$ | + | + |
| 63 | $\frac{16}{10}$ | $\frac{16}{10}$ | $\frac{30}{12}$ | $\frac{30}{15}$ | — | + |
| 63 | $\frac{15}{12}$ | $\frac{15}{12}$ | $\frac{45}{20}$ | $\frac{20}{10}$ | — | + |

* Preoperative
Postoperative

**Table 6.**  *Worksheet for Grading Subjective and Objective Function*

Please check only *one* line in the Before Surgery and Now columns for *each* of the two main categories, and return promptly in the enclosed stamped, self-addressed envelope.

| BEFORE SURGERY | SYMPTOMS (PAIN IN THE BIG TOE) | NOW |
|---|---|---|
| _____ | No symptoms; no restriction of normal activity | _____ |
| _____ | Symptoms occasional, causing no restriction of normal activity | _____ |
| _____ | Symptoms constant, causing intermittent limitation of normal activity | _____ |
| _____ | Symptoms constant, causing total limitation of normal activity | _____ |

| | MOTION OF BIG TOE | |
|---|---|---|
| _____ | Good motion (big toe up 30°, and big toe down 15°) | _____ |
| _____ | Stiffness of motion *either* up or down | _____ |
| _____ | Stiffness of motion *both* up and down | _____ |
| _____ | No movement possible | _____ |

| | YOUR OVERALL FEELING REGARDING BIG TOE | |
|---|---|---|
| | Satisfied with results | _____ |
| | Some improvement but not entirely satisfied | _____ |
| | Dissatisfied | _____ |

Would you recommend this operation to someone else with the same problem?   Yes__No__.
Additional comments:

**Table 7.** *Symptoms Relative to the Big Toe Before and After Surgery*

| AFTER SURGERY | CONSTANT SYMPTOMS—INTERMITTENT LIMITATION OF ACTIVITY* | | OCCASIONAL SYMPTOMS—NO RESTRICTION OF ACTIVITY* | | CONSTANT SYMPTOMS—TOTAL LIMITATION OF ACTIVITY* | |
|---|---|---|---|---|---|---|
| | Number | Per Cent | Number | Per Cent | Number | Per Cent |
| No symptoms; no restriction of normal activity | 7 | 63.64 | 9 | 75.00 | 1 | 100 |
| Symptoms occasional, causing no restriction of normal activity | 2 | 18.18 | 2 | 16.67 | 0 | 0 |
| Symptoms constant, causing intermittent limitation of normal activity | 2 | 18.18 | 1 | 8.33 | 0 | 0 |
| Symptoms constant, causing total limitation of normal activity | 0 | 0 | 0 | 0 | 0 | 0 |

* Before surgery.

**Table 8.** *Motion Relative to the Big Toe Before and After Surgery*

| AFTER SURGERY | GOOD MOTION (UP 30° AND DOWN 15°)* | | STIFFNESS OF MOTION EITHER UP OR DOWN* | | STIFFNESS OF MOTION BOTH UP AND DOWN* | |
|---|---|---|---|---|---|---|
| | Number | Per Cent | Number | Per Cent | Number | Per Cent |
| **Good motion (big toe up 30°, and big toe down 15°)** | 10 | 76.92 | 4 | 80 | 2 | 33.34 |
| Stiffness of motion *either* up or down | 2 | 15.38 | 0 | 0 | 2 | 33.33 |
| Stiffness of motion *both* up and down | 1 | 7.70 | 1 | 20 | 2 | 33.33 |
| No movement possible | 0 | 0 | 0 | 0 | 0 | 0 |

* Before surgery.

# CONCLUSION

A three-in-one technique has been presented for consideration in the treatment of hallux valgus in all age groups, the results being analyzed from both an objective and subjective standpoint. The indications for the procedure are outlined with favorable results for relief from pain and deformity.

# REFERENCES

1. Akin, O.F.: The treatment of hallux valgus—A new operative procedure and its results. Med. Sentinel, *33*:678-679, 1925.

2. Balacescu, J.: Un caz de hallux valgus simetric. Rev. Chir., 7:128-135, 1903.

3. Bonney, G., and Macnab, I.: Hallux valgus and hallux rigidus. A critical survey of operative results. J. Bone Joint Surg., *34B*:366-385, 1952.

4. Durman, D.C.: Metatarsus primus varus and hallux valgus. Arch. Surg., *74*:128-135, 1957.

5. DuVries, H.L.: Surgery of the Foot. Ed. 2. St. Louis, C.V. Mosby Co., 1965.

6. Giannestras, N.J.: Foot Disorders—Medical and Surgical Management. Ed. 2. Philadelphia, Lea & Febiger Co., 1973.

7. Giannestras, N.J.: Modified Akin procedure for the correction of hallux valgus. Am. Acad. Orthop. Surg., *21*:254-261, 1972.

8. Hardy, R.H., and Clapham, J.C.: Observations on hallux valgus. J. Bone Joint Surg., *33B*;376-391, 1951.

9. Heuter, C.: Klinik der Gelenkkrankheiten. Leipzig, F.C.W. Vogel, 1871, pp. 339-351.

10. Kelikian, H.: Hallux Valgus, Allied Deformities of the Forefoot and Metatarsalgia. Philadelphia, W.B. Saunders Co., 1965.

11. Loison, M.: Note sur le traitement chirurgicale du hallux valgus d'apres l'etude radiographique de la deformation. Bull. Mem. Soc. Chir., *27*:528-531, 1901.

12. McElvenny, R.T.: A study of hallux valgus; its cause and operative management. Quart. Bull. Northwestern Univ. M. School, *18*:286-297, 1944.

13. Silver, D.: The operative treatment of hallux valgus. J. Bone Joint Surg., *5*:225-232, 1923.

14. Spalteholz, W.: Hand Atlas of Human Anatomy, Vol. 2. Ed. 7. Philadelphia, J. B. Lippincott Co.

15. Truslow, W.: Metatarsus primus varus or hallux valgus. J. Bone Joint Surg., 7:98-108, 1925.

*Chapter 16*

# Diaphysectomy for Severe Acquired Overlapping Fifth Toe and Advanced Fixed Hammering of the Small Toes

MELVIN H. JAHSS, M.D.*

While many operative procedures have been described for acquired overlapping fifth toe and for advanced hammering of the small toes, the author has been disappointed in either the inadequacy of the correction or by the postoperative complications. This chapter presents a simple operation applicable for both advanced acquired overlapping fifth toe and advanced hammer toes giving excellent correction both cosmetically and functionally without any postoperative problems.

Acquired overlapping fifth toe should be differentiated from the congenital variety. In the congenital variety, which is often hereditary, the toe gradually becomes flattened side to side so that by adulthood, even if the deformity becomes fixed, it rarely results in any mechanical problems from standard commercial shoe wear obviating the need for surgery. The overlapping is more prominent in the congenital type and is associated with considerable skin and soft tissue contracture in the dorsal web space between the fourth and fifth toes. In the more pronounced cases there is a severe fixed extension contracture at the metatarsophalangeal joint but usually only a relatively mild flexion contracture at the proximal interphalangeal joint. In contrast, in the acquired type the toe hammers more than overlaps, contracts only slightly toward the fourth toe, exhibits a more severe contracture at the proximal interphalangeal joint, and develops a painful corn over the dorsolateral aspect of the proximal interphalangeal joint. The toe becomes thickened and bulbous resulting in further discomfort with shoe wear (Fig. 1). Isolated hammering of the fifth toe is seen most frequently in people having box-like rather than tapered forefeet with fat looking, short, squared-off toes of relatively equal length. In these patients the condi-

* Associate Clinical Professor of Orthopedic Surgery, Mt. Sinai School of Medicine, New York, New York; Attending and Chief of Orthopedic Foot Service, Hospital for Joint Diseases, New York, New York.

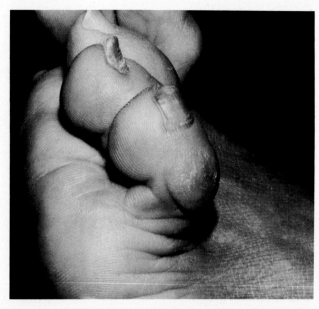

Figure 1.   Typical clinical appearance of advanced 90° to 90° acquired overlapping fifth toe.

tion is caused by the pressure and friction of the lateral side of the tapered toe box of shoes against the adjacent fifth toe.

When acquired hammering is seen in conjunction with similar hammering of the other small toes, the etiology is related to the basic cause of the generalized hammering, the commonest being forefoot equinus and cavus. In such cases one usually sees taut hypertrophied extensor tendons along with painful metatarsal calluses and inflexible metatarsal rays. Less frequently, multiple hammering of the small toes is seen in conjunction with rheumatoid arthritis, psoriasis, spinocerebellar diseases with cavus, poliomyelitis, peripheral nerve injuries, brain damage, post meningitis, and in massive trauma to the leg with or without compartment syndrome causing foot edema with secondary rigid toe contractures.

In general, multiple hammer toe deformities vary in their clinical appearance from flexible to completely rigid with varying degrees of involvement of either or all of the metatarsophalangeal, proximal interphalangeal, and distal interphalangeal joints. The type of treatment depends upon the degree of flexibility,[7] the joint or combination of joints involved, the severity of the involvement, the flexibility of the metatarsal rays, as well as the cause of the hammering. Thus a pes cavus with flexible hammer toe deformities requires only correction of the cavus to relax the tight extensors. However if the toes have become rigidly deformed surgical correction of the hammer toes as well will be required.

In cases of "frozen" toes secondary to massive trauma, peripheral nerve injuries, and spinocerebellar diseases such as Charcot-Marie-Tooth, the contractures often involve only the proximal and distal interphalangeal joints. The contractures are usually advanced and rigidly fixed with minimal or no involvement of the metatarsophalangeal joints.

While all types of hammer toe deformities occur with rheumatoid arthritis, most frequently the contractures predominate at the metatarsophalangeal joints with dorsal dislocation of the bases of the proximal phalanges over the rigidly depressed metatarsal heads. At the same time the proximal interphalangeal joints are usually fixed in mild flexion with the distal interphalangeal joints in compensable flexible hyperextension. Such cases are best treated by resection of the metatarsal heads and necks and bases of the proximal phalanges.

Early cases of hammering associated with forefoot equinus reveal mild flexible extension contractures of the metatarsophalangeal joints, similar flexible flexion contractures of the proximal interphalangeal joints, or varying degrees of both. The moderate cases show varying degrees of rigid contractures of the metatarsophalangeal and proximal interphalangeal joints. Usually one or the other contractures predominates; the surgical correction then is directed mainly toward the more severe element of the deformity. In the most severe cases the rigid extension contractures of the metatarsophalangeal joints approach 90 degrees of deformity as do the flexion contractures of the proximal interphalangeal joints. Associated changes include contractures of collateral ligaments, extensor and flexor and lumbrical tendon shortening plus subluxation at the metatarsophalangeal level. It can readily be seen from both a clinical and therapeutic point of view that the classification of hammer toes merely into intrinsic plus and intrinsic minus deformities is an inaccurate oversimplification. While fairly satisfactory procedures have been described for the mild to moderate deformities, the fixed 90 degree to 90 degree deformity remains a problem. Total or near total proximal phalangectomy results in a flail cosmetically poor looking toe. Combined procedures directed at both the metatarsophalangeal and proximal interphalangeal joints become excessively involved and may even result in aseptic necrosis of the proximal phalanges or metatarsal heads.[10] Shortening of the diaphyses of the proximal phalanges does not release any fixed joint deformities.[1]

As with hammer toes, the surgical correction of acquired overlapping fifth toe depends primarily upon the degree of hammering, the amount of soft tissue contracture, and in the more severe cases the fixed joint contractures of up to 90 degrees at both the metatarsophalangeal and proximal interphalangeal joints. Such advanced fixed contractures are resistant to soft tissue release[3, 5, 8, 12] including skin, tenotomies, and capsular and collateral ligament stripping. The modified Z plasty of Galland[2] on the tight dorsal skin may only partially release the contracture. Any attempts at a true Z plasty in this area are prone to at least partial slough with secondary extension contracture. In general, extensive soft tissue release without bone resection is both unduly traumatic and insufficient for the more advanced cases. Extensor tendon transplant[6] satis-

factorily corrects only flexible deformities, is quite an extensive procedure and may lead to slough or even partial loss of the fifth toe. As with
the other small toes, excision of the proximal half of the proximal
phalanx[11] fails to correct the deformity at the proximal interphalangeal
joint, while distal hemiphalangectomy similarly fails to correct the deformity at the metatarsophalangeal joint. Excision of the entire proximal
phalanx usually leads to a functionless floppy toe. Kelikian[4] therefore
advises proximal phalangectomy combined with syndactyly to the fourth
toe. Ruiz-Mora[9] also excises the entire proximal phalanx and stabilizes
the fifth toe quite simply by plantar skin plication. While the Kelikian
and Ruiz-Mora operations adequately correct the advanced deformities,
they involve considerable soft tissue and bone dissection. The stripping
of the joint capsules is particularly traumatic. This frequently results in
pronounced persistent postoperative swelling of the fifth toe often for as
long as nine months. In light of the above the author has preferred to
carry out diaphysectomy of the proximal phalanx, tenotomy of flexor
and extensor tendons, and plantar skin plication.

## OPERATIVE PROCEDURE

The patient lies supine with the foot near the end of the operating
table and the surgeon is seated facing the plantar aspect of the foot. No
tourniquet is used. For the fifth toe a liberal vertical ellipse of skin is removed from the plantar medial aspect of the fifth toe at the level of the
flexion crease. The ellipse includes skin from the adjacent plantar fat
pad (see Fig. 5). The slight medial shift of the skin excision is to allow
closer approximation of the fifth toe to the fourth which should preferably slightly underlap the fourth toe. By gentle blunt dissection the medial branch of the plantar digital neurovascular bundle to the fifth toe is
retracted medially and the underlying diaphysis of the proximal phalanx
will be found to lie just beneath the open wound as the bases of the plantar aspect of the toes lie at the level of the distal third of the proximal
phalanges (Fig. 2). The flexor tendon is tenotomized which also facilitates removal of the diaphysis. The diaphysis is first cut across with a thin
double action bone cutter or a needle nosed rongeur as close to its
metaphysis as possible (Fig. 3). If inadequate bone is removed the remaining nubbin of diaphysis will point dorsally. The diaphysis is then
similarly transected close to the head of the proximal phalanx. The entire diaphysis is readily removed. No capsular stripping is necessary since
the diaphysis is cut both proximally and distally just beyond the joint
capsules (Fig. 4.) A small curved clamp or a tendon hook is then used to
retract the still tight extensor tendon out of the wound and the tendon is
tenotomized. The skin is closed in a dorsiplantar direction (Figs. 5 and 6)
and a small bandage applied with the fifth toe approximating the fourth.
The entire procedure takes about five minutes. There is minimal postoperative discomfort and no significant postoperative swelling has been
encountered. Walking is commenced in about four to five days and the
sutures removed in three weeks. The toe is strapped postoperatively

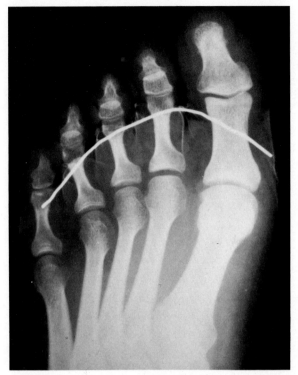

Figure 2. Roentgenogram of foot with wire placed over plantar aspect of base of toes.

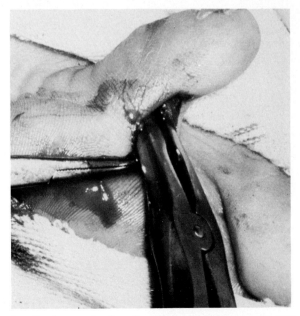

Figure 3. Cutting proximal portion of diaphysis of proximal phalanx.

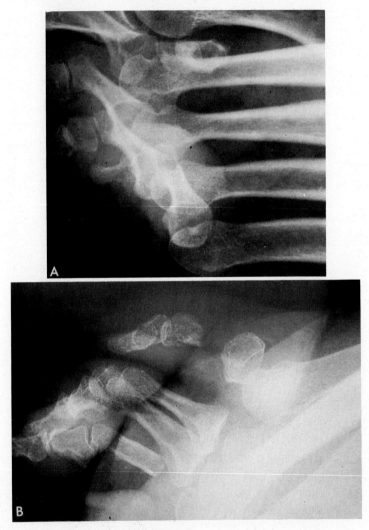

Figure 4.   *A*, Preoperative lateral roentgenogram of the foot seen in Figure 1. *B*, Postoperative lateral roentgenogram.

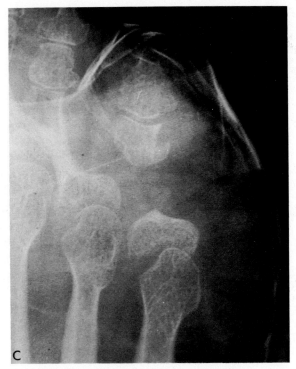

Figure 4 (*Continued*). *C*, Postoperative anteroposterior roentgenogram.

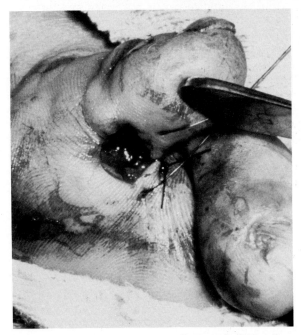

Figure 5.   Skin closure. Note extent of removal of skin ellipse.

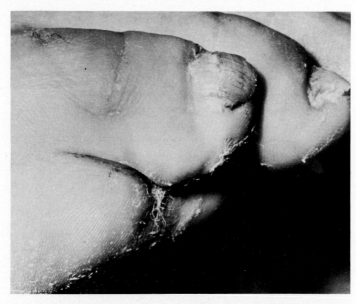

Figure 6.   Appearance of patient's foot in Figure 1 two weeks postoperatively.

every week until it stabilizes in its corrected position which may take three to five weeks.

For the advanced hammer toe deformity of the second, third, and fourth toes (Fig. 7A) a similar ellipse of plantar skin is removed at the base of the toes and adjacent fat pad and the diaphysectomy is performed as on the fifth toe. The toes, by retaining the proximal and distal ends of the proximal phalanges, do not unduly shorten nor become unstable (Fig. 7B). In cases of multiple corrections it may be necessary to make vertical skin incisions to avoid producing too narrow a skin flap between adjacent ellipses (Fig. 8). Postoperatively the toes are strapped at weekly intervals in slight overcorrection until stabilized.

When the 90 degree to 90 degree deformity involves only the proximal and distal interphalangeal joints, the diaphysectomy and tenotomies are performed on the middle phalanx through a midline lateral incision. These patients often have poor subcutaneous padding with very thin tense atrophic skin encasing the toes. This mandates delicate soft tissue nonhandling carefully hugging the diaphysis to strip off the often adherant overlying skin.

## RESULTS AND CONCLUSIONS

Of the diaphysectomies performed over the past seven years, there has been one partial recurrence of multiple hammer toe deformities as-

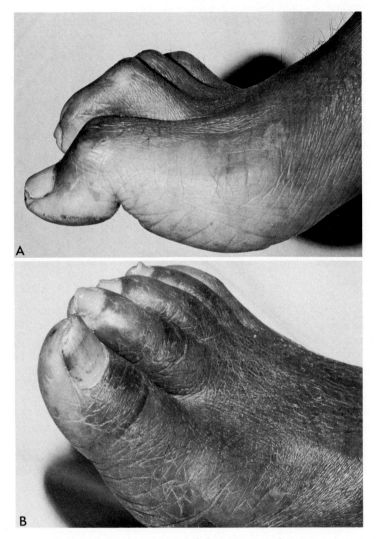

Figure 7. *A*, Multiple rigid hammer toe deformities secondary to massive trauma of the leg. *B*, Appearance of the foot seen in 7*A* six months postoperatively.

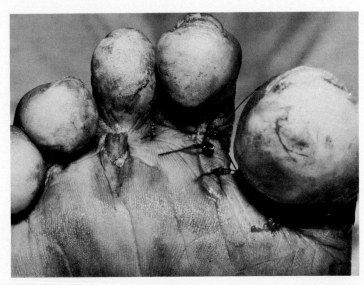

Figure 8.   Note vertical plantar incision under second toe and diaphysis being delivered from incision under third toe. The distal end was transected first to facilitate mobilization of the diaphysis.

sociated with massive leg trauma and partial sciatic nerve damage including paralysis of the toe flexors. The recurrence was due to resumption of function of the extensor tendons which had been tenotomized during the operative procedure. The tenotomies were repeated and a more radical ellipse of plantar skin was removed maintaining the correction to date.

The author has designed a simple operation for advanced hammering of the small toes where the hammering is associated with rigid contractures of both the metatarsophalangeal and proximal interphalangeal joints of up to 90 degrees. The operation consists of a diaphysectomy of the proximal phalanx, flexor and extensor tenotomies, plus plantar skin plication. For the more uncommon combined advanced deformities of the proximal and distal interphalangeal joints the diaphysectomy is performed on the middle phalanx through a midlateral incision.

All patients have been satisfied with both the cosmetic and functional results. There have been no complications such as sloughs or infections except for one recurrence which was readily rectified.

## REFERENCES

1.  Bragard, K.: Die Beseitigung der Hammerzehe durch juxtakapitale Resektion aus der Grundphalanx. Zeit. Orthop. Chir., 47:283, 1926.

2. Galland, W. I.: Operation for correction of congenital overlapping of fifth toe. Bull. Hosp. Joint Dis., *1*:93, 1940.

3. Goodwin, F. C., and Swisher, F. M.: The Treatment of congenital hyperextension of the fifth toe. J. Bone Joint Surg., *25*:193, 1943.

4. Kelikian, H., Clayton, L., and Loseff, H.: Surgical syndactylia of the toes. Clin. Orthop., *19*:208, 1961.

5. Lantzounis, L. A.: Congenital subluxation of the fifth toe and its correction by periosteocapsuloplasty and tendon transplantation. J. Bone Joint Surg., *22*:147, 1940.

6. Lapidus, P. W.: Transplantation of the extensor tendon for correction of the overlapping fifth toe. J. Bone Joint Surg., *24*:555, 1942.

7. Parrish, T. F.: Dynamic correction of claw toes. Orthop. Clin. North Amer., *4*:97, 1973.

8. Royle, N. D.: The treatment of dorsal displacement of the little toe. Med. J. Aust., *1*:560, 1934.

9. Ruiz-Mora, J.: Plastic correction of overriding fifth toe. Orthop. Letters Club, *6*:1934.

10. Scheck, M.: Degenerative changes in the metatarsophalangeal joints after surgical correction of severe hammer-toe deformities. A complication associated with avascular necrosis in three cases. J. Bone Joint Surg., *50A*:727, 1968.

11. Scrase, W. H.: The treatment of dorsal adduction deformities of the fifth toe. J. Bone Joint Surg., *36*:146, 1954.

12. Wilson, J. N.: V-Y correction for varus deformity of the fifth toe. Brit. J. Surg., *41*:133, 1953.

# Chapter 17

# The Enigma of
# Morton's Neuroma

VIRGIL R. MAY, JR., M.D.*

The patient with acute paroxysms of burning pain in the forefoot has been treated with many different therapeutic regimens for relief and cure over the past years. The first recorded description of this entity was published in 1845, "Treatise on Corns, Bunions, the Diseases of the Nails and the General Management of the Feet" by Lewis Durlacher, chiropodist to the Queen.

At that time the condition was thought to be an affection of the digital nerves. "Another form of neuralgic affection occasionally attacks the plantar nerve on the sole of the foot between the third and fourth metatarasal heads, but nearest the third and close to the articulation with the phalanx. The pain which cannot be produced by the mere pressure of the finger, becomes very severe while walking or whenever the foot is put to the ground."[13]

T. G. Morton,[22] whose name the disease bears and who is generally credited with first describing it, called it "a peculiar and painful affection of the fourth metatarsophalangeal articulation." He explained the etiology on the basis that the heads of the first three metatarsals are nearly in a line and are less movable than the remaining ones. The head of the fourth is a quarter of an inch behind that of the third. At their anterior extremities the fourth and fifth metatarsal bones are very mobile. When the transverse arch is compressed, the head of the fifth metatarsal bone and its proximal phalanx come directly into contact with the head and neck of the fourth metatarsal bone; consequently the digital nerves are compressed or pinched. While this anatomical explanation seemed to suffice in the case of the fourth and fifth metatarsals, it failed to explain metatarsalgia originating around the heads of the second and third bones.

During this time various names for the condition began to appear. Luxation podalgia was suggested by Dana.[5] Anterior metatarsalgia was introduced by Pollosson[25] who postulated the condition to be the result of a certain laxity of the transverse metatarsal ligament which permitted a partial infraction of the arch whereby the third metatarsal phalangeal

---

* Clinical Professor of Orthopedic Surgery, Medical College of Virginia, Virginia Commonwealth University, Richmond, Virginia.

articulation became dislocated downward compressing the nerves. Morton's theory contended that the branches of the lateral plantar nerve were involved because of a slight luxation of the metatarsophalangeal joint of the third and fourth toes.

It was Thomas S. K. Morton[23] who actually gave the disease its credited name of "Morton's toe" or "Morton's painful affection of the foot." His work vividly described the symptoms of six patients and upheld the etiologic explanation of the older Morton. Others who endorsed Morton's causative exploration were Woodruff,[32] Guthrie,[10] and Bradford.[3] Once the luxations were reduced by massage, the pain ceased.

Goldthwait[9] was a strong advocate of the theory that obliteration of the anterior transverse arch was the direct cause of paroxysmal anterior metatarsalgia. Stern[29] observed the "almost all patients suffering from this affliction will be found to belong to the better and wealthier classes. Very few had sedentary occupations and almost all elicited the history of a severe trauma shortly before the pain first came on; runaway accidents, jumping into the saddle, football, tennis and the like are given as the causative agent of the trauma."

Whitman[31] concluded that "depressions of the anterior arch predispose to pain because of the weakness of its muscles and its ligaments." If the relaxation of the ligaments allowed one metatarsal to fall below its adjacent member then lateral pressure would cause the pain. He attributed the cause of the condition to be weakness and thought that the shoe was the most important predisposing factor because of its weakening effect upon the natural support of the foot. It was claimed that his patients were relieved of pain by the insertion of a metal foot plate in the shoe.

No mention of resection of the nerve had been made until during a meeting of the Philadelphia Academy of Surgery in March of 1893.[24] Thomas S. K. Morton, after presenting a paper on Morton's painful affection of the foot, answered a question raised as to whether the painful nerve rather than the joint or toe might be excised.He responded that there would be difficulty in finding the nerve and that unless all the soft parts surrounding the joint were removed, some branches would remain. He further stated that he felt the pain was a result of the peculiar relation of the fourth joint, as compared with the third and the fifth joints, and that no treatment other than joint removal would be of value.

Other operations advocated during this time for the nonresponsive conservative cases were amputation of the toe, cauterization, insertion of a heated needle at the pain site to destroy the nerve, and hypodermic injection of carbolic acid.[17] Even in more recent times, alcohol was injected into the fourth and fifth space with a subsequent sloughing of the skin and intervening tissues.[18] Nevertheless, the typical burning and throbbing pain subsided after scarring of the wound, which may have taken three to six months, had occurred.

Resection of the digital nerve leading to the fourth and fifth toes was first suggested by Mills[21] but it is unknown whether this procedure had actually been carried out. It was categorically stated by Betts[1] that the lesion is a "neuritis of the fourth digital nerve with a pronounced neuroma in all cases." He also explained the mechanics of stretching without compressing the nerve. A longitudinal plantar incision and neurectomy were carried out in 10 patients, followed by resection of the nerve. McElvenny[20] described the technique of a dorsal web bisecting incision of the nerve that was generally carried out.

## SYMPTOMS

Most writers describe Morton's toe as a severe throbbing, burning pain on the plantar and dorsal surface of the forefoot involving the general area between the third and fourth toes of one of the feet. It may involve the metatarsal cleft between the second and third metatarsals.

Patients variously describe their pain as "sickening, like treading on something hot, as if walking on hot coals or having a hot burr between the toes on walking." The patients have severe paroxysms of burning pain.[7, 8, 16, 19, 27, 30] The pain, as a rule, results from walking, but occasionally may also result from irritation of bed sheets, putting on shoes and socks, or some other insignificant manipulation. The longer the symptoms have persisted, the more radiation, proximally on the the dorsal surface, seems to be noted. The pain may reflect up the anterior ankle and tibial portion of the lower leg to the knee. Paresthesia into the third and fourth toes is commonly experienced. If the intrametatarsal space is involved at another location, the pain and paresthesia will involve the adjacent toes. The pain is further described as sharp, penetrating, and boring with increasing intensity (Fig. 1). The soreness persists for several hours, or two to three days following an attack. Changes in temperature, particularly from warm to cold, may trigger the pain.

One of the most characteristic statements by the patient regards the experiencing of an irresistible desire to remove the shoe on the affected foot and to massage and flex the toes. Most patients do not complain of generalized foot discomfort, disability, or fatigue, other than the time when pain is present.

## PHYSICAL FINDINGS

No significant structual abnormalities in the feet and legs are noticed, which many lend a clue to the etiology. Generally there is an absence of corns, excessive callous formation, hammer toes, or other lesions of the feet or legs. Even during an attack in a patient, I have not observed vasomotor changes in the forefoot, such as cyanosis, redness, swelling, or sweating. The foot has a normal appearance. The most consistent physical finding is tenderness on firm palpation between the metatarsal heads, and proximally, at least to the junction of the middle and upper third of the metatarsal shaft in the involved cleft. Occasionally a feeling of fullness is present on the dorsal surface of the foot between the involved metatarsal cleft. Rarely a snapping of the fourth phalangeal metatarsal joint is observed on compression of the forefoot.

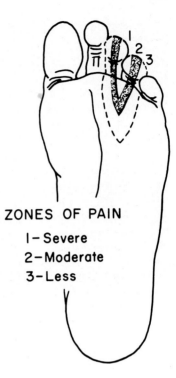

Figure 1.   The pain is more severe along the digital nerve distal to the lesion.

**ZONES OF PAIN**

1 – Severe

2 – Moderate

3 – Less

## THE BASIC LESION

The lesion usually is a yellowish white mass located just anterior to and between the heads of the metatarsals. Generally it is approximately 2 cm. in length. With pressure by fingers between the metatarsal heads on the plantar surface of the sole, quite often a pearly white, flattened or fusiform mass is elevated into the wound (Fig. 2). This somewhat resembles an amputation neuroma. The mass is encapsulated by pearly white connective tissue. The distal and proximal ends of the digital nerve are normal in circumference. In most patients the specimen shows a reddish brown discoloration at the ends of the nerve, a result of hemorrhage at the sides of the excised nerve. The tumor mass involves the bifurcation of the digital nerve. The plantar nerve fibers are seen traversing throughout the mass of fibrous collagen-like material. These fibers give the patient a sensation that his foot is thickened.

## OPERATIVE TECHNIQUE

Most studies refer to the operative incision as being made on the plantar surface of the foot. The author believes this plantar scar to be

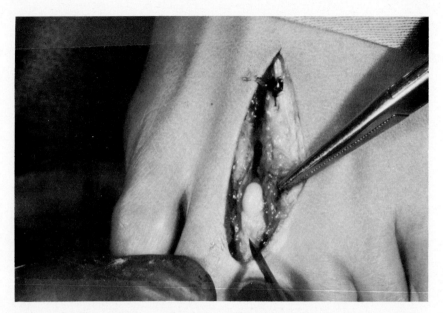

Figure 2.    Finger pressure on the plantar surface elevates the lesion into clear vision.

bothersome in weight bearing. A combination dorsal and plantar incision, which extended into the web space between the metatarsal heads,
was advocated by Cohen.[4]

More recently Kaplan[12] has advocated a transverse plantar incision
at the base of the toes just proximal to the interdigital folds. This takes
longer to heal and should infection occur, a large weight bearing portion
of the forefoot would be involved and the resulting scar tissue would be
in the direct center of weight bearing.

The dorsal incision extends 1½ inches to the web of the toes. The
subcutaneous tissue is incised between the metatarsal heads. No exposure
of the phalangeal metatarsal joint is necessary, nor are the extensor
tendons exposed through their sheaths. The transverse metatarsal ligament is seen and incised. The transverse adductor hallucis may be seen
lying deep in the wounds.

Elevation of the mass exposes the normal digitations traversing to
each side of the toes. These digitations are excised distally, and the lesion
then is freed from its distal end (Fig. 3). By lifting the lesion upward with
gentle traction, generally a few adhesions are seen binding the lesion
against the capsule and adventitious tissue. The lesion is mobilized and
dissected well proximal to the metatarsal heads and then removed.

## HISTOPATHOLOGY

The classic anatomic researches of Key and Retzius[14] established years ago the prevailing conception of the structure of a peripheral nerve.

These investigations named three supporting structures of sheaths beside the sheath of Schwann with which each nerve is provided. Bundles of nerve fibers are bound together by an endoneurium, being distinct from the loose connective tissue. Several neural fasciculi are held together by the epineurium.

Injuries to peripheral nerves have been classified by Seddon[28]—as neuropraxia, axonotmesis, and neurotmesis. In lesions of minor severity in which axons are injured and their function is only temporarily disrupted, lack of wallerian degeneration is commonly caused by pressures or blows of minor severity. This condition is known as neuropraxia.

Axonotmesis implies loss of axone function without structural damage at the site of injury and some wallerian degeneration in the distal nerve segment. The connective tissue sheaths of the nerve remain intact or are only slightly damaged. There is little or no true neuroma formation. The most common causes of such lesions are bruising, continuous pressure of long duration, or attrition.

The classification neurotmesis comprises nerve injuries in which whole or part of the nerve is severed including its endoneurium and

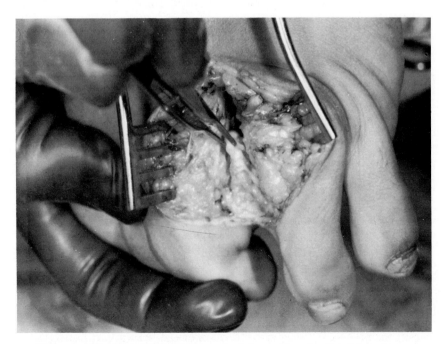

Figure 3.   The lesion is detached anteriorly by excising the digital branches.

perineurium, but not necessarily all of the epineurium. Such lesions often form true neuromas.

I conceive the Morton toe lesion as falling into the first two categories. The longer duration of symptoms determines whether axonotmesis prevails.

Many investigators have reviewed the effects of pressure and related trauma to peripheral nerves elsewhere in the body, but only a few have investigated the plantar digital nerve lesion experimentally.

Stretching of peripheral nerves was done in experiments by Denny-Brown and Doherty.[6] In gentle kneading of a nerve, intraneural hemorrhage was induced and within a few days rapidly resolved with complete return of function, leading to some fibrosis. There was no evidence of hemorrhage or inflammatory reaction encountered even in the patient with acute, recently acquired symptoms; however, fibrosis was quite evident. By increasing the stretching forces they observed that the peroneal nerve of a cat extended rather easily and retracted to its original length except when attempting to double the length. It was then noted that the nerve remained redundant in its new length with swelling, hemorrhage, and later thrombosis of the vessels with fibrosis. Ischemic lesions and patchy necrosis were observed in the more severely stretched nerves. Inflammatory cells were also present in the cat nerves.

From these experiments it appears that as with the plantar digital nerves, the axons and their myelin sheaths are extensible. However the nerves are limited by the perineurium and epineurium. Elastic tissue was abundant in the blood vessels but only sparsely scattered in the proliferated connective tissue of the lesion (Fig. 4). Changes in the interstitial connective tissue of nerves as in a chronically bruised nerve show a progressive increase in collagen, associated with thickening of the endoneurial tubules and reduction in their caliber. In regeneration of the nerve fibers their size depends to a large extent on the character of the nerve fibers from which they arise as well as the state of the distal tubules.[11]

Later King[15] reported the pathologic findings in five tumors. He indicated the tumors were not true neoplasms as seen in neuromas but represented a "reactive hyperplasia" with sclerosing and degenerative changes. He termed the lesion "sclerosing neuroma" to distinguish this group from the usual amputation or traumatic neuroma.

Eighteen cases, 16 in women and two in men, were recorded in 1947 by Bickel and Dockerty.[2] The most common and earliest nerve change found was interstitial edema associated with irregular demyelinization and swelling of the entire nerve trunk. Marked proliferation of the Schwann cells gave an appearance of increased cellularity.

Microscopic specimens from 31 patients with the clinical diagnosis of Morton's toe have been examined by the author. These specimens were stained with Harris hematoxylin and counterstained with eosin. The cytoplasm, collagen, and connective tissue stain a bright transparent pink, the nuclei a blue-black. The most constant finding was abundant proliferation of perineural connective tissue. This proliferation appeared to reflect itself in increased numbers of Schwann cells and later degeneration of Schwann cells. The proliferation of connective tissue ex-

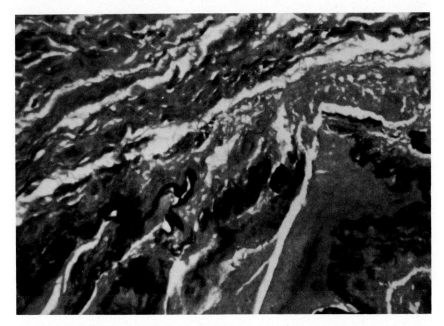

Figure 4.   Morton's toe lesion is shown in a tangential cutting demonstrating abundant elastic fibers of an arteriole staining black. There are no elastic fibers in the abundant surrounding fibrous tissue. (Verhoeff's stain. × 175.)

tended around the main nerve and between its branches. In the true lesions, there was not only proliferation of the connective tissue elements, but even hyaline degeneration. The lesions quite often showed very dense fibrous connective tissue with an increase in capillary formation.

Bodian's method (protargol silver albumose) was used for staining nerve fibers. This was difficult but successful in the larger lesions. In these the axons were frequently separated by excess fibrous tissue (Fig. 5). Some of the axons were edematous and many showed degeneration.

In the Wilder silver stained material, the reticulum stained violet to black. When the perineurium and epineurium were thickest with a large amount of collagen within the nerve bundles, the silver stain failed to exhibit nerve fibrils although some may have been present among the slightly impregnated connective tissue fibers (Fig. 6). Similar impregnations are true neuromas or normal nerve in which both thick and thin axons were readily demonstrable.

Elastic tissue in the nerves was observed as the digital nerves are stretched in push-off. This material was abundant in the arterial walls, but there were scant amounts found in the nerve lesions (Fig. 7). Morton lesions show only relatively few nerve bundles as compared with other neuromas. No small bundles were seen without perineurium.

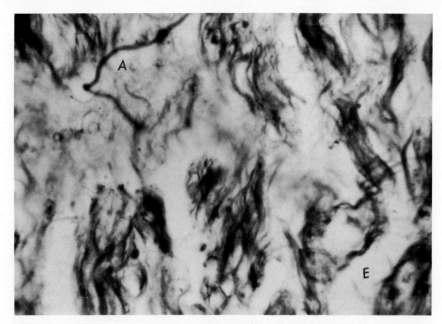

Figure 5. A longitudinal section of a fascicle of an old Morton's toe lesion. Marked degeneration is seen in the axons. One axon is distorted, thickened with its nucleus (*A*). The proliferated endoneural connective tissue is extremely edematous (*E*). Nerve filaments and a Schwann cell have bypassed a large vacuole. The numerous bundles of amyelinated axons are embedded in the connective tissue. (Bodian's stain. × 400.)

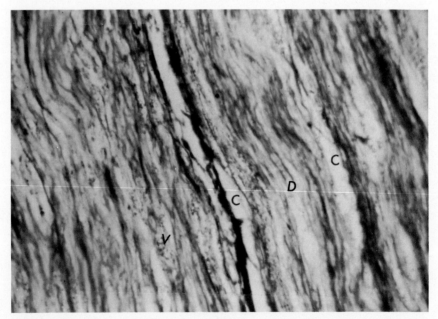

Figure 6. A longitudinal section of a Morton's toe lesion shows a large amount of collagen within the nerve bundles (*C*). Degenerating myelinated fibers are shown (*D*). Some edematous connective tissue is seen (*C*). Vacuoles are present within some of the tubules (*V*). Few Schwann cell nuclei are seen. (Wilder's silver stain. × 350.)

230

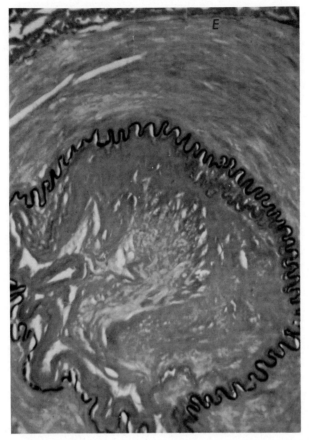

Figure 7.    There were scant amounts of elastic tissue throughout the lesion (*E*). The elastic fibers stain black. (Verhoeff's ferric chloride stain. × 200.)

Fibrosis is much increased in the diseased specimens as compared with the normal nerve specimens. Because of lack of cellular elements, these lesions cannot be classified as true neoplasms. Hyalinization of the perineurium was frequently found.

The lesions in early stages showed a proliferation of Schwann cells (neurinoma). Later a neurofibroma with marked hyperplasia of the connective tissue elements increased sclerosis and proliferation of vessels. There is severe degeneration of the nerve bundles in the mature lesion.

## DISCUSSION

Even as late as 1963, the degenerative lesion of the nerve was thought to be secondary to vascular disease. Mechanical injury to the vasorum of the artery reflects degenerative changes. In sections taken from the normal foot in patients 30 to 60 years of age, the arteries and arterioles showed thickening of the subintimal layer caused by hyperplasia of the tunica elastica and media. The arterial changes vary in different sections of the same specimen. In none of the vessels were there atheromatous intimal changes or calcifications. The lumen of the vessels, both in the lesion and normal digital nerves, had become irregularly constricted and even obliterated. In some specimens the remaining lumen was filled with a fibrous mass and in some recanalization of the lumina was attempted. No inflammatory infiltration of the vessels was encountered. The swollen arteries in the intraneural type seemed unchanged as a rule. However, in some of the pathological specimens there seemed to be proliferation of intraneural capillaries.[26]

From these observations of normal specimens exhibiting the same degenerative vascular changes as specimens with lesions, it can be concluded that this was a normal process of the foot resulting from aging and the pressures of walking and standing upon the gradually thinning sole treads. Endarteritis appeared to occur with the same frequency here as in the diseased nerves.

A combination of anatomical features and biomechanical stresses contribute to the formation of Morton's toe syndrome. The fourth and fifth metatarsals are more mobile in the "take-off" position of the foot. This mobility is reflected in spreading the metatarsal heads lateralward. The pressure on the metatarsal heads in the "take-off" position is four times greater than the pressure in the "standing balanced" position. This may be increased readily by the slightest shift in the thrust of the tibia on the talus.

Contraction of the intrinsic muscles of the foot is present during phasic activity of the foot; thus any hypertrophy of the transverse adductor hallucis could cause an increase in pressure on the digital nervers.

When the toes dorsiflex in the "push-off" position, the digital nerves are stretched under the unyielding transverse metatarsal ligament. The plantar aponeurosis which is stretched around the metatarsal heads would also tend to increase pressure on the affected digital nerve. The neuritis arises in the first place from minor constant trauma, the third and fourth metatarsals taking most of the weight on the outer side of the foot.

The sole of the foot thins, diminishing in protective lobules with age, This causes the nerves to be more vulnerable to pressures from the floor, particularly when walking on uneven surfaces.

These intrinsic factors all contribute to the formation of Morton's neuroma. When enlarging fibrosis begins, the nerve is immobilized still further. Edema causes further enlargement of the nerve. It then becomes apparent that function and age are not alone sufficient to constitute all the factors responsible for this disease.

The most common extrinsic factor producing injury to the foot is footwear. In walking in shoes with high heels, the body weight is thrust forward on the ball of the foot. Since no relation has been made to the heels, the arch and the shank of the shoe are unbalanced, placing continous strain on the foot. On a mechanical basis it is understandable how foot disorders develop.

Fashion of shoes has frequently assumed a more prominent role than comfort in shoe manufacturing. The changes in design have been made mostly in the shape of the toe section. The variations have included open, round, square, and oval toes of varying widths and lengths. The width of the shoe and its sole across the anterior ends of the metatarsals is most important. Most shoes tend to constrict the normal spreading of the metatarsals and interfere with proper contraction of the plantar muscles. This reduces stability causing interference with the dynamics of the forefoot. This constriction may also produce congestion with edema about the metatarsophalangeal joints, which results in secondary changes in the restricted plantar nerve lying between the metatarsal heads.

This lesion is not a true neoplasm. The microscopic appearance, anatomy and biomechanics of the foot point definitely to traumatic neuritis with proliferation of connective tissue elements. It is a reactional, irritative fibrosis of the connective tissue elements surrounding the nerve trunks and should be classified as a neurofibroma.

## REFERENCES

1. Betts, L. O.: Morton's metatarsalgia: Neuritis of the fourth digital nerve. Med. J. Aust. *1*:514-1515, 1940.

2. Bickel, W. H., and Dockerty, M. B.: Plantar neuromas, Morton's toe. Surg. Gynecol. Obstet., *84*:111-116, 1947.

3. Bradford, E. H.: Metatarsal neuralgia or Morton's affection of the foot. Bos. Med. Surg. J., *2*:52, 1891.

4. Cohen, H. H.: Morton's metatarsalgia, Bull. Hosp. Joint Dis., *13*:206-211, 1952.

5. Dana, C. L.: The acro-neuroses (functional nervous affections of the extremities. Med. Rec., *28*:85-87, 1885.

6. Denny-Brown, D., and Doherty, M.D.: Effects of transient stretching of peripheral nerve. Arch. Neurol. Psychiat., *54*:116-129,1945.

7. Dieterle, J. O., and Kuzman, J. R.: A case of Morton's metatarsalgia (Morton's toe), treated by operation. Wisc. Med., J., *45*:967-968, 1946.

8. Fett, H. C., and Pool, C. C.: Plantar interdigital neuroma or Morton's toe. Am. J. Surg., *78*:522-525, 1949.

9. Goldthwait, J. E.: The anterior transverse arch of the foot: Its obliteration as a cause of metatarsalgia, Bos. Med. Surg. J., *131*:233-234, 1894.

10. Guthrie, L. G.: On a form of painful toe. Lancet, *1*:628, 1892.

11. Gutman, E., and Sanders, F. K.: Recovery of fiber numbers and diameters in the regeneration of peripheral nerves. J. Physiol. *101*:489-517, 1943.

12. Kaplan, E. B.: Surgical approach to the plantar digital nerves. Bull. Hosp. Joint Dis., *11*:96-97, 1950.

13. Kemp, C. E.: Morton's metatarsalgia. Brit. Med. J., *1*:1005, 1949.

14. Key, A., and Retzius, G.: Studien in der Anatomi des Nerversystems und des Bindergrivebes. Stockholm, Norstedt Ach. Soner, 1876.

15. King, L. S.: Note on the pathology of Morton's metatarsalgia. Am. J. Clin. Path., *16*:124-128, 1946.

16. Kite, J. H.: Morton's toe syndrome. J. Med. Assoc. Ga., *36*:309-313, 1947.

17. Lange, F.: Zur Behandlung der "Tarsalgie." Munsch Med. Wochenschr., *45*:258-260, 1898.

18. Lapidus, P. W., and Wilson, M. J.: Morton's neuralgia. Bull. N. Y. Med. Coll., *12*:34-46, 1949.

19. Lewin., P.: The Foot and Ankle. Ed.2. Philadelphia, Lea & Febiger, 1941.

20. McElvenny, R. T.: The etiology and surgical treatment of intractable pain about the fourth metatarsophalangeal joint (Morton's toe). J. Bone Joint Surg., *25*:675-679, 1943.

21. Mills, C. K.: Pain in the feet. J. Nerv. Ment. Dis., *13*:3-20, 1888.

22. Morton, T. G.: Peculiar and painful affection of the metatarsophalangeal articulation. Am. J. Med. Sci., *71*:35-45, 1876.

23. Morton, T. S. K.: Metatarsalgia (Morton's painful affection of the foot) with an account of six cases cured by operation. Ann. Surg., *17*:680-699, 1893.

24. Morton, T. S. K.: Metatarsalgia (Morton's painful affection of the foot). Ann. Surg., *17*:718-719, 1893.

25. Pollosson, A.: Anterior metatarsalgia. Lancet, *1*:436-553, 1889.

26. Ringertz, N., and Unander-Scharin, L.: Morton's disease (a clinical and pathoanatomical study). Acta Orthop., *19*:327-348, 1950.

27. Sayle Creer, W.: Metatarsalgia or painful forefoot. Clin. J. (London), *76*:47-53, 1946.

28. Seddon, H. J.: Three types of nerve injury. Brain, *66*:238-288, 1943.

29. Stern, W. A.: Morton's painful disease of the toes. Am. Med. J., *7*:221-225, 1904.

30. Venturi, R.: Metatarsalgia di Morton. Chir. Organi. Mov., *49*:327-339, 1960.

31. Whitman, R.: Anterior metatarsalgia. Trans. Am. Orthop. Assoc., *11*:34-53, 1898.

32. Woodruff, C. E.: Incomplete luxations of the metatarsophalangeal articulations. Med. Rec., *1*:61-62, 1890.

*Chapter 18*

# Neuropathic Foot in the Diabetic Patient

RICHARD L. JACOBS, M.D.*

Ulcers on the sole of the foot or over other areas that sustain pressure from the shoe are common in the diabetic patient (Fig. 1). These may or may not be associated with neuropathic (Charcot) joints in the foot (Fig. 2). If the ulcer is directly associated with damaged joints, the radiographic changes are sometimes improperly attributed solely to osteomyelitis or pyogenic arthritis. In most instances, however, the primary etiology for the soft tissue and skeletal lesions is diabetic neuropathy.

It has been estimated that as many as 35 per cent of all diabetic patients, regardless of adequacy of treatment of the diabetic condition, develop some degree of neuropathy. These patients are prone to develop the complications of arthropathy and perforating ulcers (mal perforant). In Martin's series of 150 diabetics with neuropathy, nine had Charcot joints and 18 had mal perforant.[20] Both these lesions are consistently underdiagnosed and failure of recognition often leads to failure of treatment of the foot lesions. Indeed, a recent study described two diabetic patients who had amputations for ulcerated draining feet. Histologic study revealed no changes in either small or large vessels to explain the development of these ulcers. With recognition and proper treatment amputation probably could have been avoided.[34] It is important not to confuse this group of problems with lesions that are primarily the result of circulatory insufficiency and that may develop in areas which are not necessarily subjected to much trauma. In general we have found that relatively conservative forms of treatment will give satisfactory results in neuropathic feet if only the diagnosis is made!

## HISTORICAL ASPECTS

Neuropathy in diabetics was described by Rollo[21] as early as 1790 and in the following years such authors as Sandmeyer,[29] Williamson,[35] Pryce,[28] Schweiger,[30] and Woltman[40] did detailed autopsies and studies of

---

* Professor and Head, Division of Orthopedic Surgery, Albany Medical College, Albany, New York.

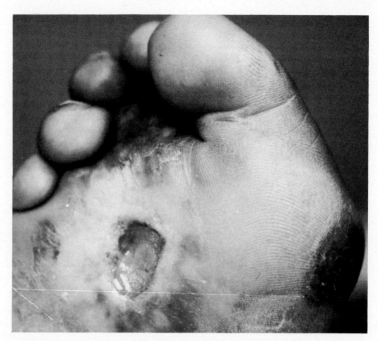

Figure 1.   Neuropathic ulcer (mal perforans) in a diabetic patient.

pathological material from diabetics. They all clearly showed degenerative changes in both the spinal cord and peripheral nerves, especially in the posterior columns of the cord and in the posterior roots. In the same era, Williamson[36-39] first described some common clinical forms of diabetic neuropathy. Sir William Osler[25] gave a superb description of a clinical case which he termed "diabetic tabes."

Of course the first clinical description of neuropathic arthropathy was of that found in tabetics which was reported by Jean Martin Charcot in a lecture to his students at the Salpetriere in 1868.[5] With all of the attention that was focused on diabetic neuropathy, it is very surprising that neuropathic arthropathy in diabetics was not recognized until Jordan[12] reported a case involving the ankle in 1936. Even today many clinicians still fail to make the connection between neuropathy, arthropathy, and perforating ulcers in their diabetic patients. Even as additional reports of this clinical entity were accumulating, some were to cling for a time to the notion that the joint changes seen in the feet of diabetic patients were a result of infection[10] and were not neuropathic. They failed to consider feet that had no associated ulceration to account for infection or joint destruction.

Most physicians now recognize neuropathy as common in diabetics and realize that neuroarthropathy is not uncommon. Most cases involve the foot and ankle, though involvement of other joints such as the knee [7, 18, 27, 31, 33] and spine [3, 14, 41] have been reported.

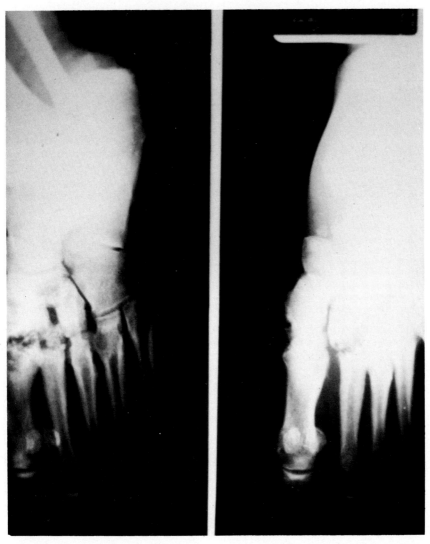

Figure 2.    Ulcers on the foot in the diabetic patient may be associated with neuropathic (Charcot) joints in the foot.

## CLINICAL FEATURES

The typical clinical presentation of diabetic neuropathy is seen in a patient who may or may not have diabetes under good control and who has stocking hypesthesia of the lower extremities. There may be decreased proprioception and pallesthesia. Deep tendon reflexes in the lower extremities are diminished or absent in over half of these patients. Motor weakness is less frequent than sensory disturbance and can be a result of primary myopathy rather than secondary to neuropathy. Complaints of paresthesia or even hyperesthesia are common. Early in the course diabetic neuropathy is especially apt to affect nonmyelinated pain fibers[22] and leads to the classic situation seen in neuropathic arthropathy of whatever etiology; relatively normal motor strength is preserved in a structure which has impaired ability to appreciate pain.

Diabetic patients with neuropathy seem to be more prone to develop plantar callosities, especially beneath the metatarsal heads. If there are claw toes, hammer toes or hallux rigidus, such callosities can appear on the plantar surfaces of the toes also. In a foot with normal sensation, when such callosities become sufficiently large they cause pain and the patient will trim them or alter gait to avoid weight bearing in the area.

In contrast, the neuropathic foot will not be as painful and full weight bearing without treatment continues. When enough callus accumulates, it acts as a hard, fixed foreign body beneath the weight bearing surfaces of the foot (Fig. 3). With time and neglect, the apex of this cornified material will cause a full thickness ulceration in the underlying dermis, even though the surface of the foot appears to be covered with a normal layer of cornified epidermis. Eventually, exudate from the ulcer bed dissects to the surface and drainage commences. If the corn is shaved or pulled away, the fully formed ulcer will be seen. To emphasize, this is characteristically on the plantar surface of the foot or toes, though ulcers can form elsewhere on the foot as with poorly fitting shoes. These plantar ulcers usually appear in the same locations that Charcot believed were the maximum weight bearing areas of the foot. Foot problems in the diabetic patient often involve both feet in a short time and early attention is important.[1]

Though microangiopathy of diabetes may be present to aggravate the situation, the *original* problem is one of deficient sensation and local pressure, not originally one resulting from impaired circulation in the foot. A patient with such a perforating ulcer may well show good pedal pulses, good color of the foot, and no gross evidence of circulatory impairment on a macroscopic level. Cases which do have badly impaired circulation (Fig. 5) may start with a neuropathic ulcer and eventuate in gangrenous change in the toes. Presumably this is because the ulcer becomes secondarily infected causing local thrombosis of already diseased small vessels. Again, early attention is important; secondary gangrene, unlike neuropathic ulceration,[22] cannot be healed!

If the neuropathic ulcer remains untreated, it may extend to bone which becomes secondarily infected. The whole problem is then often misconceived of as "osteomyelitis"; vague statements are made concern-

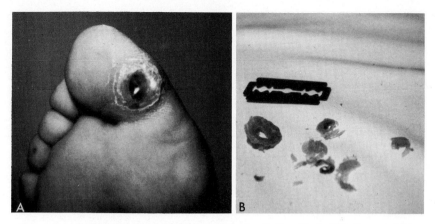

Figure 3. *A*, Hallux rigidus with plantar callosity. *B*, Cornified epithelium excised.

ing poor circulation and the susceptibility of the diabetic patient to infection. To reiterate, all of these statements may well be true, but they are not the main factors which caused the original ulceration. If the basic problem is not realized, there can be no rational prevention or treatment.

Although the ulcer may or may not be associated with any change in bone or joints, about 50 per cent of all diabetic patients with plantar ulcers will have associated neuroarthropathy of the foot.[20] There are commonly neuropathic changes in the metatarsophalangeal joint or in the toe immediately adjacent to the ulcer. Although both hypertrophic (Fig. 6*A*) and atrophic forms (Fig. 6*B*) are seen, the atrophic form is far more common in diabetic patients.[28] As with the ulcer, these bone changes may cause little or no pain, though in early stages may cause moderate discomfort. These bone changes may be modified by infection but nonetheless are chiefly neuropathic in nature. Further there are often

Figure 4. Ulcer underlying the callosity.

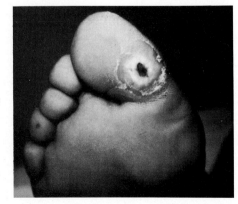

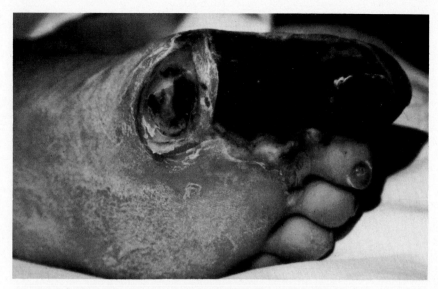

Figure 5.   Neuropathic ulcer beneath first metatarsal head with secondary infection, eventuating in gangrene of great toe.

neuroarthropathic changes elsewhere in the foot or ankle that are not associated with ulceration and will give even greater strength to this diagnostic impression.

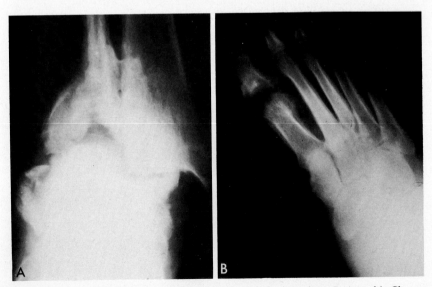

Figure 6.   *A*, Hypertrophic Charcot joint in a diabetic patient. *B*, Atrophic Charcot joint in a diabetic patient.

Arthropathy of the foot is often manifested by a diffuse thickening of the forefoot as with involvement of Lisfranc's joint or by marked effusion and deformity around the hindfoot and ankle (Figs. 2 and 7). When the subtalar joint is involved, increasing eversion of the foot at the subtalar joint causes increasing valgus of the foot and prominence of the head of the astragalus in the medial arch. As the arch flattens, ulceration may appear over the newly weight bearing astragalar head (Fig. 8). Increasing flatfoot deformity in the diabetic patient should make obvious the presence of arthropathy.

Arthropathy is claimed to be more common in the poorly regulated, longstanding cases of diabetes.[18] It has been claimed that the progress of this bone disease is arrested in at least 60 per cent of patients when adequate control of diabetes is achieved.[19] Others such as Peterson[26] claim that arthropathy progresses even in their patients in whom control of diabetes is good.

Although the arthropathy in a patient with diabetes is usually less severe and more easily controlled than that seen in a patient with syphilis, it may occasionally progress just as rapidly and cause marked destruction.[19] Opinions vary widely as to whether or not good therapeutic control of diabetes will lessen vascular and neurologic complications. A typical study found that diabetic patients with the best control of their

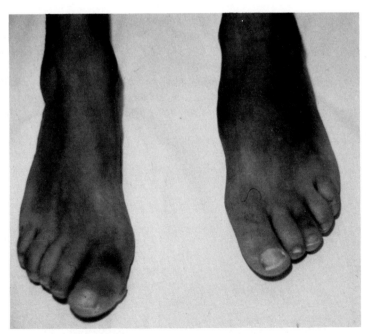

Figure 7. Diffuse thickening of left forefoot with neuroarthropathy of Lisfranc joint.

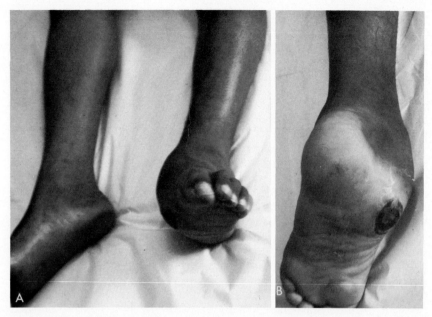

Figure 8. *A*, Diabetic flatfoot in a patient with subtalar neuroarthropathy. *B*, Ulceration beneath head of talus in the same foot.

metabolic condition have less frequent and less severe vascular lesions than those with poor control.[15] Neuropathy is at least in part related to vascular lesions of neural tissue.

Suppose then that the patient has a neuropathic foot with either arthropathic changes, perforating ulcer, or both. If there is appreciable circulatory impairment as a complication, this will adversely affect the results in the patient with ulceration and secondary infection.

With vascular disease there will be any of a number of signs or symptoms such as complaints of cold feet, foot pain at rest, claudication, color changes on dependency or elevation of the foot, decreased or absent pulses, loss of hair, thin atrophic skin with pigmentary change, and gangrenous changes which may be strictly localized. All of these can be a result of disease of the large artery and are not necessarily caused by microangiopathy. A diagnosis of microangiopathy is necessarily one of exclusion.

Pedal pulses may exist in the face of major arterial occlusion if there are adequate collaterals. An exercise test may be helpful in detecting this. The patient is walked to the point of tolerance and the pulses are again palpated. The pulse will weaken or disappear as blood flow is diverted to the dilated capillary bed in the proximal muscles. Because of this possibility, a few vascular surgeons recommend arteriography even when pedal pulses are present in the ulcerated or gangrenous foot.

If pulses can be palpated, such techniques as plethysmography, oscillometry, and use of ultrasound Doppler flowmeters do not give additional information concerning the adequacy of the capillary bed.[4] They are, however, valuable as a "noninvasive" form of evaluating the overall adequacy of blood flow in the extremity and are inexpensively and easily accomplished.

In the absence of pedal pulses, arteriography done well and completely is indicated. This should be accomplished with multiple injections to demonstrate as much of the outflow as possible. This "invasive" technique will give an anatomic picture localizing the impairment of circulation in the major vessels, but does involve some risk.

Capillary microcirculation can be severely impaired even in the presence of adequate peripheral pulses, whereas in other instances the reverse may be true.[8] A study of 52 diabetic patients showed that 46 of them had characteristic basement membrane hypertrophy and endothelial proliferation in arterioles of the lower extremity.[24] Microangiopathy may well be even more common than is usually realized, but may not be severe enough to cause clinical problems.

## TREATMENT

The best treatment of any of the lesions we have discussed is to prevent them in the first place! Any physician giving medical care to a diabetic patient should always include an examination of the feet at each visit and periodic foot and ankle roentgenograms should be obtained if this appears to be advisable. Excessive callus in pressure areas should be shaved by the physician at periodic intervals and the patient is advised to use a pumice stone to efface the callus in the interval.

The plantar surfaces of the toes in hallux rigidus and hammer toes may undergo excessive weight bearing during the push-off phase of gait and plantar callus formation and ulcers may occur here as well as in areas shown in previous illustrations. Here, as in the ulcers beneath the metatarsal heads, well placed metatarsal pads can effectively ease the pressure areas and are much more effective than metatarsal bars on the soles of the shoes.[23]

More severe cases which do not respond to such conservative measures are treated surgically before neuropathic complications can develop. Keller bunionectomy is carried out for hallux rigidus and decompressive proximal interphalangeal fusions for claw toes. The Ruiz procedure is sometimes alternatively used for claw toes. After any of these procedures metatarsal pads are still used to relieve the additional weight stress which is newly transferred to beneath the metatarsal heads.

## CLINICAL EXPERIENCE

When the patient presents with plantar ulceration of recent onset, vigorous treatment should be initiated immediately, as neglect will compound the problem in short order. The patient in Figure 9 had a fifth ray resection elsewhere for an ulcer beneath the fifth metatarsal head. He subsequently wore no protective footwear and presented with ulceration beneath the fourth metatarsal head (Fig. 9*A*) and with destruction of the fourth metatarsophalangeal joint (Fig. 9*B*). For personal reasons he did not remain for treatment at that time. Two weeks later he returned with a huge new ulcer (Fig. 9*C*). The ulcer was debrided and the patient

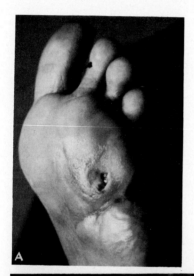

Figure 9. *A*, Mal perforans under fourth metatarsal head. Fifth ray resection for same problem in past had been carried out. *B*, Fourth metatarsophalangeal joint was destroyed.

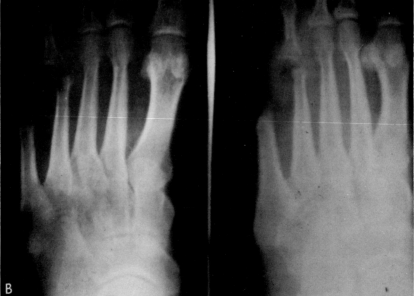

was placed on bedrest with the foot elevated. Two weeks later the ulcer was rapidly closing (Fig. 9D).

A smaller, more superficial ulcer may often be treated with an ambulatory method. Another patient had a plantar ulcer of four years' duration (Fig. 10A) with destruction of the metatarsophalangeal joint (Fig. 10B), stocking hypesthesia, and loss of deep tendon reflexes. The callus was debrided, revealing the ulcer (Fig. 10C). There was no obvious deep infection. A ½ inch sole was cut from Aliplast and directly placed on the sole of the foot. Over this, a short leg walking cast of plastic* was applied. The patient was then allowed partial weight bearing with this light weight waterproof cast. This cast and the foot may be lavaged with water if the odor of secretions from the ulcer becomes a problem. The cast will dry again overnight. The cast was removed at three weeks, and the ulcer was healed (fig. 10D) for the first time in four years. The patient was fitted with oxfords with Aliplast insoles and was able to achieve full weight bearing. Examination at six months (Fig. 10E) showed that the ulcer had remained well healed and there was no progression of the arthropathy. With such treatment, superficial ulcers almost always close rapidly.

In patients with a deep, perforating ulcer that is associated with secondary infection of bone and joint, we have discarded much of our early pessimism and usually attempt local treatment of the ulcer rather than ray resection or amputation as primary treatment, unless there is overwhelming infection or circulation in the foot is grossly and obviously impaired. As was shown earlier, ray resections can shift the pressure to

---

* Lightcast II; Merck, Sharpe and Dohme, West Point, Pennsylvania.

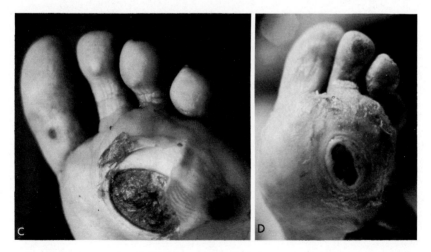

Figure 9 (Continued). C, Rapid progression of ulceration in still another site on the same foot, two weeks later. D, Rapid healing after two weeks of bed rest.

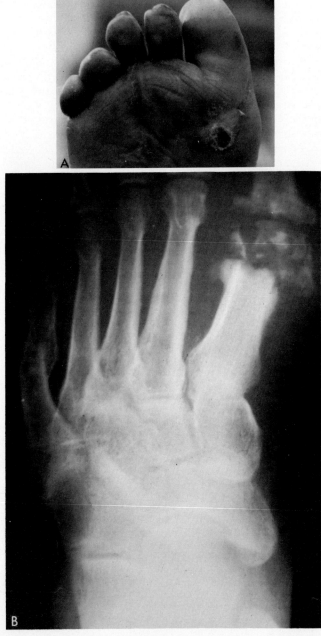

Figure 10. *A*, Superficial perforating ulcer and callus. *B*, First metatarsophalangeal joint was destroyed.

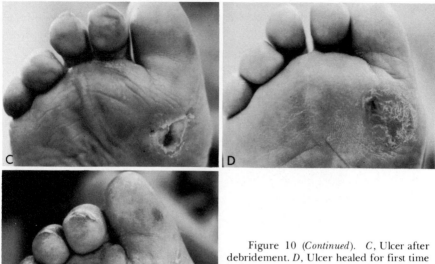

Figure 10 (*Continued*). *C*, Ulcer after debridement. *D*, Ulcer healed for first time in four years. *E*, Ulcer remains healed at six months with protective shoeing.

another metatarsal head where the whole problem may occur again unless foot care is maintained. Further it should always be kept in mind that amputation of one leg in a diabetic patient is followed by loss of the other leg in about one third of patients within three years.[14]

Local treatment of the deep ulcer almost always should be attempted. This ulcer (Fig. 11*A*) was present for about two years and was undermined for about 1 inch around its entire margin. The first metatarsophalangeal joint (Fig. 11*B*) was completely destroyed. The ulcer was widely debrided along with underlying bony prominences (Fig. 12*A*) to leave a shallow walled crater. This removed a large amount of relatively avascular infected tissue (Fig. 12*B*). The tip of a small plastic catheter was placed into the cavity and fluffs were packed over this. An appriopriate topical antibiotic solution was slowly dripped over the ulcer bed for several days and discontinued when the wound appeared grossly clean. Systemic antibiotics were continued along with bedrest. Good granulations were apparent by the fifth postoperative day (Fig. 12*C*) and split thickness grafts were applied. In such a case, the cavity is not directly weight bearing, so that the difficulties of a pedicle graft can be avoided by the use of the free grafts. The take was nearly 100 per cent (Fig. 12*D*),

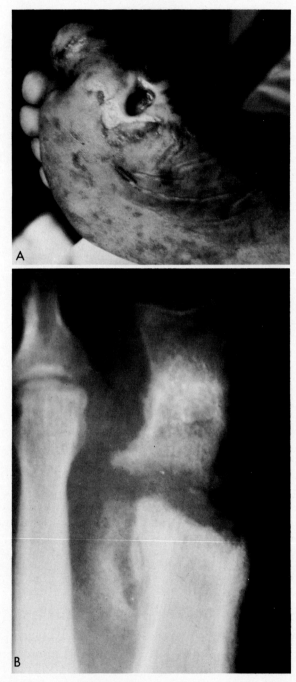

Figure 11. *A*, Deeply undermined mal perforans of two years' duration. *B*, Destruction of first metatarsophalangeal joint.

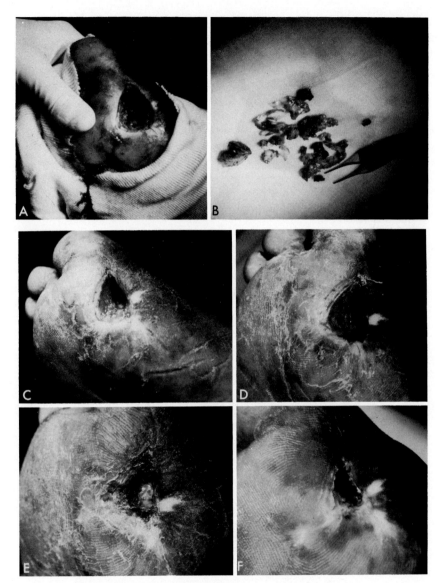

Figure 12. *A*, Shallow cavity remaining after debridement. *B*, A large amount of tissue was debrided. *C*, Good granulations were seen by the fifth postoperative day. *D*, Nearly 100 per cent take of split-thickness skin grafts. *E*, Forefoot edema subsided and cavity shrank. *F*, Protective shoeing was applied when healing was complete.

forefoot edema rapidly subsided, and the cavity shrank (Fig. 12*E*). Protective shoeing was applied when healing was complete (Fig. 12*E*). In this instance, a surgical boot with an Aliplast insole has served well. This energy-absorbing material helps to prevent recurrence of the ulcer resulting from further trauma. Aliplast, however, tends to pack down with time and usually must be changed at intervals of about two to three weeks if it is to remain effective. After two to three such changes, we use a more durable sponge rubber.

If there is major vessel disease, consultation with a vascular surgeon is indicated. If there are good pulses and microangiopathy appears to be a complication, early amputation of gangrenous toes associated with plantar ulcers may well be successful and should be attempted. This patient (Fig. 13) had successful amputation of two toes on separate occasions and his plantar ulcers healed. Consideration should always be given first to partial amputations of the foot.[16, 32] The old dictum of below-knee amputation for any gangrenous change in the foot of a diabetic patient can no longer be supported.

If the foot is pulseless, however, healing after such amputation may be poor. In these instances, the value of bypass grafts for the patient with proximal occlusive disease is well established and the use of femoropopliteal bypass grafts can almost be called routine. Fairly recent developments in vascular surgery should now be considered for the patient with distal occlusive disease. The diabetic patient will sometimes have occlusion at or below the popliteal trifurcation. The recently developed technique of long femorotibial bypass grafts may restore a pedal pulse and be conclusive in partial salvage of the foot. In some instances

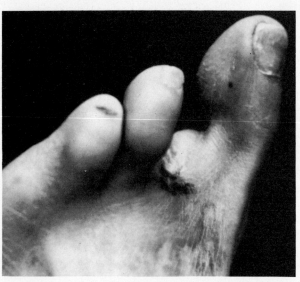

Figure 13.   Local amputations are often successful.

this has even obviated the need for partial amputation.[9] It should be noted that these enthusiastic reports are limited to vascular surgeons who have carried out a relatively large number of the procedures. Results have been less striking for others.

## Neuropathic Arthropathy

What more regarding arthropathy in the feet of diabetic patients? Johnson has made a much-needed and most important series of observations[11] concerning neuropathic arthropathy that echo the thoughts expressed by Virchow and von Volkmann so many years ago. Equally qualified authorities since their time have failed to state these principles forcefully enough.

Neuropathic joints and spontaneous fractures involving bone or joint are the results of trauma to insensitive structures. As with any other bone or joint fracture or injury, they will heal completely if they are given the chance. The older literature contains many reports of healing of fractures, resorption of joint effusion, and tightening of previously lax ligaments when the injured member is rested for a sufficient time to allow healing to predominate over new destructive changes. Adequate and prolonged immobilization will give healing the best chance to occur. The injured area must be rested for a much longer time than is necessary in a normal individual with a similar injury. Immobilization, preferably in plaster, continues until effusion subsides, until the extremity is no longer warm as compared with the other normal side (indicating that the injury and repair process with its inflammatory process is close to completion), and until secure healing of the injury is seen on roentgenograms.

As Charnley[6] has emphasized, it is next to impossible to immobilize forefoot injuries adequately in plaster, especially if weight bearing is permitted. Nonetheless, we do use nonweight bearing short leg casts when forefoot arthropathy is involved as this at least partially immobilizes the forefoot.

Aftercare when immobilization is discontinued emphasizes continuing protection of the foot and ankle against extremes of motion. A double-upright brace with fixed ankle joint is used in instances of ankle or subtalar involvement. Less commonly a molded leather lacer with steel stays is worn inside a surgical boot. Such forms of bracing or shoe modifications must be checked at intervals to prevent progression of the neuropathic changes.

There is no doubt that with proper treatment, arthropathy can be arrested in diabetic patients and will cause little trouble other than that associated with residual secondary deformity of the foot.[22] These are some telling reasons for the practice of preventive medicine and conservative surgery in diabetic patients with neuropathic feet.

The concept of preventive medicine may soon pursue interesting new lines. It has been claimed that the drug Clofibrate (ethyl chlorophenoxyisobutyrate) may be effective in the treatment of peripheral neuropathy in diabetic patients[2] and seven of nine patients in one study showed decreased paresthesias and numbness, increased strength, and return of deep tendon reflexes. We have no experience with this form of therapy.

Of course the ultimate form of treatment of diabetes and avoidance of its complications may lie in such heroic measures as pancreatic allo-transplantation, which has been tried over 30 times in humans without remarkable success. An implantable "black box" biomechanical analogue of the pancreatic islets is under development at the University of Southern California. New ideas are not lacking in research of this important disease.

## REFERENCES

1. Baddeley, R. M. and Fulford, J. C.: A trial of conservative amputations for lesions of the foot in diabetics. Brit. J. Surg., 52:38, 1965.

2. Berenyi, M. R., Straus, B., and Miglietta, O. E.: Treatment of diabetic neuropathy with clofibrate. J. Am. Geriat. Soc., 19:763, 1971.

3. Brain, W. R.: Diseases of the Nervous System. Ed. 4. London, Oxford University Press, 1951, p. 812.

4. Burgess, E. M., Romano, R. L., Zettl, J. H., et al.: Amputations of the leg for peripheral vascular insufficiency. J. Bone Joint Surg., 53A:874, 1971.

5. Charcot, J. M.: Sur quelques arthropathies qai paraissant dépendre d'une lesion du cerveau on de la moelle épiniere. Arch. Physiol. Norm. Pathol., 1:161, 1868.

6. Charnley, J.: The Closed Treatment of Common Fractures. Ed. 3. Baltimore, The Williams & Wilkins Co., 1963.

7. De Takats, C.: The peripheral neurovascular lesions in diabetics. Proc. Am. Diabetes Assoc., 5:183, 1945.

8. Dunlop, C. R.: Problems of ischemia in the lower extremities. New Engl. J. Med., 246:219, 1952.

9. Guilmet, D., Soyer, R., Gandjbakhch, I., et al.: Distal femoro-tibial bypass. J. Cardiovasc. Surg., 37:478, 1971.

10. Hodgson, J. R., Pugh, D. G., and Young, H. H.: Roentgenologic aspect of certain lesions of bone: Neuropathic or infectious? Radiology, 50:65, 1948.

11. Johnson, J. H. T.: Neuropathic fractures and joint injuries. J. Bone Joint Surg., 49A:1, 1967.

12. Jordan, W. R.: Neuritic manifestations in diabetes mellitus. Arch. Int. Med., 57:307, 1936.

13. Jordan, W. R.: Effect of diabetes on the nervous system. South. Med. J., 36:45, 1943.

14. Kahan, M., and Chafison, Y. J.: The diabetic foot. Hosp. Med., 9:15, 1972.

15. Keiding, M. R., Root, H. F., and Marble, A.: Importance of control of diabetes in prevention of vascular complications. J. A. M. A., 150:964, 1952.

16. Kritter, A. E.: A technique for salvage of the infected diabetic gangrenous foot. Orthop. Clin. North Am., 4:21, 1973.

17. Lewis, R. W.: The Joints of the Extremities. Springfield, Charles C Thomas, 1955.

18. Lippmann, E. M., and Crow, J. L.: Neurogenic arthropathy associated with diabetes mellitus. J. Bone Joint Surg., 37A:971, 1955.

19. Martin, M. M.: Charcot joints in diabetes mellitus. Proc. Roy. Soc. Med., 45:503, 1952.

20. Martin, M. M.: Diabetic neuropathy. A clinical study of 150 cases. Brain, 76:594, 1953.

21. Martin, M. M.: Involvement of autonomic nerve fibers in diabetic neuropathy. Lancet, 1:560, 1953.

22. Martin, M. M.: Neuropathic lesions of the foot in diabetes mellitus. Proc. Roy. Soc. Med., 47:139, 1954.

23. Milgram, J. E.: Office measures for relief of the painful foot. J. Bone Joint Surg., 46A:1095, 1964.

24. Moore, J. M., and Frew, I. D.: Peripheral vascular lesions in diabetes mellitus. Brit. Med. J., 2:19, 1965.

25. Osler, W., and McCrae, T.: The Principles and Practice of Medicine. New York, Appleton-Century Crofts, 1920, p. 429.

26. Petersen, A.: Arthropathia diabetica. Acta Orthop. Scand., 30:217, 1960.

27. Pryce, T. D.: On diabetic neuritis, with a clinical and pathological description of three cases of diabetic pseudo-tabes. Brain, 16:416, 1893.

28. Rodnan, G. P.: In Hollander, J. L. (Editor): Arthritis and Allied Conditions. Ed. 7. Philadelphia, Lea & Febiger, 1966, p. 1111.

29. Sandmeyer, W.: Beitrag zur pathologischen anatomie des diabetes mellitus. Deutsch Arch. F. Klin. Med., 50:381, 1892.

30. Schweiger, L.: Uber die tabiformen veranderangen der hinterstrange beim diabetes. Arb. Neurol. Inst. Wein Univ., 14:391, 1908.

31. Shore, T. H. C.: Diabetic neuropathy. Letter to the editor. Lancet, 2:738, 1947.

32. Smith, A. G., and Casingal, E. L.: Management of diabetic patients with foot lesions. Surg. Gynecol. Obstet., 128:85, 1969.

33. Spear, G. E.: Diabetic arthropathy (letter to the editor). Lancet, 2:963, 1947.

34. Strandness, D.E., and Bell, J. W.: A comparative evaluation of peripheral arterial disease in the diabetic and non-diabetic. Rev. Surg., 22:77, 1965.

35. Williamson, R. T.: Changes in the posterior column of the spinal cord in diabetes mellitus. Brit. Med. J., 1:398, 1894.

36. Williamson, R. T.: On the knee jerks in diabetes mellitus. Lancet, 2:138, 1897.

37. Williamson, R. T.: Note on the tendo Achillis jerk and other reflexes in diabetes mellitus, Rev. Neurol. Psychiat., 1:667, 1903.

38. Williamson, R. T.: Changes in the spinal cord in diabetes mellitus. Brit. Med. J., 1:122, 1904.

39. Williamson, R. T.: The symptoms due to peripheral neuritis or spinal lesions in diabetes mellitus, Rev. Neurol. Psychiat., 5:550, 1907.

40. Woltmann, H. W., and Wilder, R. M.: Diabetes mellitus: Pathologic changes in spinal cord and peripheral nerves. Arch. Int. Med., 44:576, 1929.

41. Zucker, C., and Marder, M. J.: Charcot spine due to diabetic neuropathy. Am. J. Med., 12:118, 1952.

*Chapter 19*

# Work-Related Injuries of the Foot and Ankle

BARNARD KLEIGER. M.D.*

Work-related injuries are a serious problem in this country. Statistics vary as to the frequency of such injuries, depending upon the agency compiling them. The National Safety Council[1] reported that in 1971 there were 2,300,000 disabling, compensable injuries, and this figure excludes work-related injuries not covered by compensation.

The cost in dollars is, of course, exorbitant — about 9.3 billion dollars — and a shockingly small percentage of this sum goes to the injured worker for wage compensation and medical costs. About two thirds of the money is used for fire losses, the money value of time lost by workers other than the injured worker, the cost of investigating accidents, writing reports, and insurance administrative costs.[1]

This book is concerned with injuries of the foot and ankle, and again, according to the National Safety Council, in 1971 there were 230,000 injuries to the foot and toes. Injury to the ankle is included in the 300,000 leg injuries. Since ankle injuries are more frequent than all other lower limb injuries combined,[3] it would not be amiss to assign half or 150,000 of these to the ankle. Therefore, about 380,000 or roughly 16.5 per cent of accidents involve the foot and ankle.

## OCCUPATIONAL DISEASE

In this book occupational injury is discussed; however, as physicians, occupational disease is also our concern. The 1969 New York State Report of Compensated Cases Closed[5] defined occupational disease as that resulting from the nature of employment and comes about as a "natural incident, creating a hazard in excess of the hazard attending employment in general." It seems strange that in a state as large as New York only 28 workers had conditions that met this definition for occupational diseases of the lower limbs as compared with the 25,742 compensable injuries to the lower limbs. Many people work at jobs that require long periods of standing on hard

---

* Attending Orthopedic Surgeon, Hospital for Joint Diseases, New York, New York; Clinical Professor, Mt. Sinai School of Medicine, New York, New York; Visiting Professor, Albert Einstein College of Medicine, Bronx, New York.

surfaced floors. As we all know, some of these workers develop foot pain without injury and others develop pathological changes in response to such repeated trauma.

## STATISTICAL INFORMATION

The anatomical terminology used in reports studied[1, 2, 4, 5, 7] was not standardized. Most important, the statistics are broken down by industry and there is no information that reveals what the worker was doing at the time he was injured. If better preventive measures are to be developed, it is essential to know all the circumstances of an accident.

Furthermore, all the statistics lose significance because no baseline is provided — the number of people employed or the number of man hours worked is not given.[6]

### Compensable Injuries in Actor's Equity Union

To determine how statistical information can be used to evaluate causes of injury, I reviewed the compensable injuries sustained by members of Actors' Equity. Actors' Equity is a small union of 19,000 members, including all varieties of performers — actors, dancers, singers, and so forth. During the past four and one-half years, there were 321 compensable injuries, of which more than one third (119) involved leg, ankle, foot, or toes. Of the 119 there was sufficient information to study 107 injuries.

Ninety-one injuries were sustained during a performance. In 19 it could not be determined whether the injured person was performing or not and three were definitely not performing.

The nature of the accident was unclear in 30 of the 107 injuries. In 20 the patient twisted his foot and ankle. Eighteen performers were injured on impact with another performer or with an object on the stage. Fifteen were injured in falls, nine on stairs, and seven performers tripped on a defective stage floor. Five were hurt in jumps, and in three instances something was dropped on the performer's foot.

These accidents suggest a great deal but much information is still lacking. We know that while at work a performer is intent. The lighting or lack of it may obscure other performers or objects on stage, especially during entrances and exits. If lighting were improved, if performers and props were more carefully placed, and if stairs and floors were in good condition, injuries could be reduced.

The diagnosis in eight of the 107 patients suggested occupational disease rather than injury. Three patients had skin problems attributed to dancing barefoot. The other conditions were induced by chronic strain or were results of an injury.

These injuries caused periods of disability ranging from one day to a period of 52 weeks of total disability with a permanent partial disability. The latter injury very probably ended the actor's career.[7]

## CONCLUSION

It is to be hoped that compensable injury statistics will be changed from a mere score card to a determination of causes and effects. Such a change could bring about preventive measures that might reduce the occurrence of these injuries. Also, a detailed study of occupational disease is warranted.

### ACKNOWLEDGMENTS

I am grateful for the assistance of Ms. Jennie Spadafora of the National Safety Council, Chicago, Illinois; to Mr. John Pupo of the State of New York Workmen's Compensation Board, New York, New York; and to Ms. Helene Tetrault of Actors Equity, for providing statistical material.

## REFERENCES

1. Accident Facts. National Safety Council, 1972, pp.23-39.

2. California Work Injuries, 1969. Department of Industrial Relations, Division of Labor Statistics and Research, September 1970, Table 12.

3. Ciccone, R., and Richman, R.: A report of injuries encountered in parachute training in air borne troops at Ft. Benning, Ga. during World War II. J. Bone Joint Surg. 30A:77, 1948.

4. Compensable Work Injuries in Pennsylvania, 1969. Department of Labor and Industry. Bureau of Research and Statistics, November 1970, Table 16.

5. Compensated Cases Closed, 1969. New York. Workmen's Compensation Board. Bulletin 24, p. 4.

6. Ludwig, E. G., and Collette, J. C.: Some misuses of health statistics. J.A.M.A., 216:493, 1970.

7. Tetrault, H.: Personal communication, 1973.

*Chapter 20*

# Treatment of Fractures of the Forefoot in Industry

VERNER S. JOHNSON, M.D.*

Except for the detailed work of McKeever[11] in 1944, there are few written studies regarding treatment of fractures of the forefoot. An occasional article has appeared about metatarsal fractures but most of the discussion has been brief and confined to textbooks. Here, treatment has been similar and repetitive.

Historically, Lewin[9] thought most metatarsal fractures and some "bedroom fractures" of the phalanges should be treated by traction and banjo splint until callus was evident.

Key and Conwell[8] believed "these fractures should be treated seriously; unless accurate reduction and firm union in the correct position is obtained, prolonged disability may result." They recommend a short leg cast be applied or else "production of exuberant callus with resultant pain on weight bearing will result. Early motion and weight bearing are usually to be avoided."

Watson-Jones[12] felt equally stongly that a "walking plaster be kept in place until union is sound." He felt that fractures of the necks of one or more metatarsal bones cause serious disability if displacement is not reduced.

Textbook after textbook repeats essentially the same treatment for fractured metatarsals—closed reduction and plaster fixation, or open reduction if the correction cannot be maintained. It is repeatedly stressed that prevention of shortening and correction of deformity is mandatory. In general a short leg boot cast with gradual ambulation has been consistently recommended. Patients have responded well to these time-tested methods of treatment. However, orthopedic literature lacks statistical studies as to morbidity. On the other hand, almost paradoxically, over the last decade particularly, orthopedic literature is abundant with articles challenging treatment of the metatarsals and phalanges by wedging, shortening, rotation, excision of joints, excision of one or more metatarsal heads, and total excision of the entire metatarsal bone. These varied foot conditions include plantar keratoses[5] and other causes of

* Associate Professor of Orthopedic Surgery, University of Massachusetts School of Medicine, Worcester, Massachusetts; Chief of Orthopedic Surgery, The Memorial Hospital, Worcester, Massachusetts.

metatarsalgia,[4] such as rheumatoid arthritis, plantar warts, overlapping toes, claw toes, splay foot, bunionettes, and Frieberg's disease. Here too, these patients have benefited from time-tested methods. It would appear that somewhere between these two extremes must lie the logical way to treat fractures of the metatarsals and toes.

This chapter suggests that fractures of the forefoot have probably been overprotected and overtreated in the past. Fractures of the phalanges require only sensible emergency care, protective splinting usually to the next member toe, symptomatic medication, and immediate ambulation. Closed metatarsal fractures necessitate immediate compressive support and immediate ambulation followed by early semirigid support of the foot and continued ambulation. Open reduction is rarely necessary and can be limited to open or closed fractures with complete and irreducible displacement.

At the onset, it should be understood that the fractures discussed are not associated with fracture dislocations of the tarsometatarsal joints. The hazards of these have been clearly defined by Granberry, Liscomb,[7] Gissoni,[6] and others.[3]

## METHOD AND SELECTION OF CASES

A composite study of 350 consecutive patients with forefoot fractures is presented. The first group is a retrospective analysis of 250 patients with 287 fractures of the forefoot. These have been collected over a 15 year period at a manufacturing plant in central Massachusetts. This company of 5,000 employees has a self-sufficient hospital with equipment for x-ray films, a full time medical director, and multiple part time physicians.[1] The author served as an orthopedic consultant and personally reviewed all the charts and x-ray films of the patients presented, but did not initiate treatment on all the patients. The method of treatment was not original with the author but was adopted because of the success of early ambulation with semirigid support rather than with the use of a rigid plaster cast.

It was the policy of the company that a patient with a plaster cast, or external support such as crutches or a cane, cannot work in the actual manufacturing area because of the potential hazard to himself and others.

After orthopedic consultation, in the absence of open fractures or fractures with complete displacement, usual procedure includes giving patients first aid, ice packs, and medication for symptoms. The feet are elevated, dressings are applied, and several pairs of fluffy socks are provided. Patients are carefully fitted with an oversized snug-fitting work shoe and allowed to go back to their regular job or adjusted work if necessary. If they felt unable to do their work, they were provided with a crutch (preferably one) or a cane, a supporting shoe, and allowed to stay home until symptomatically improved. Immediate ambulation and weight bearing on the fractured foot (herein lies the key) was encouraged. Oral medication for pain was given freely (Fig. 1).

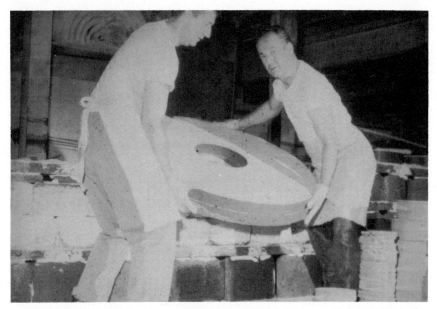

Figure 1.   Heavy and awkward objects that are repetitively handled manually are the most frequent causes of crushing injuries of the forefoot. At least 70 per cent of fractures would probably be prevented if a properly fitted safety cap shoe were worn.

Patients with open or grossly displaced fractures were treated in the appropriate manner in a local hospital. In fractures of the distal metatarsals, where the distal head fragments were displaced toward the sole of the foot, closed manipulation was first attempted under anesthesia in the operating room and was usually successful. The reduction was accepted if the fragments were in any degree of apposition and not displaced toward the sole. Shortening was usually accepted particularly in single or multiple fractures of the middle three metatarsals. The unacceptable reductions were then treated, under the same anesthesia, with appropriate heavy Kirschner pin intramedullary fixation and the ambulatory routine started as with the closed fractures.

The second group of patients is a comparable series of 100 consecutive patients (with 113 fractures) collected in cooperation with an insurance company.[2] These are exclusive of the patients treated at the manufacturing company. They were treated by various members of the orthopedic and surgical community by various methods.

These two groups have been compared as to treatment, morbidity, number of days of disability, amount of compensation and medical expenses paid, and the wages lost per employee. These two groups are then further compared as to the cost to the employer, the insurer, and the employee and the actual cost intercalated between the two groups. The distribution of fractures in the forefoot was essentially the same as the industrial group.

## DATA

As outlined in Figure 2, the distribution of the fractures is 50 per cent in the large toe ray, 25 per cent in the small toe ray, and nearly 25 per cent in the middle three rays combined.

The loss of time resulting from the various fractrues is as outlined in Table 1. It was noted that the majority of the fractures were incurred in the medial and lateral portions of the foot and most of them in the phalanges. In brief, 243 (85 per cent) of the fractures presented are of the phalanges. Only 20 patients (8 per cent) lost time from work because of the phalangeal fractures.

One of the prolonged cases (and the only female patient) was a slightly displaced fracture of the first phalanx of the fourth toe (Table 1). She was apprehensive and difficult, refusing the usual method of ambulatory treatment and was subsequently treated by her own physician with a plaster cast. She remained out of work for 12 weeks and was one of the two patients with Sudeck's atrophy in the series. The other prolonged case was an undisplaced fracture of the proximal end of the second metatarsal. He was also treated with a non-weight bearing plaster cast for four weeks and then ambulated in a walking cast. He was out of work for 14 weeks. X-ray films taken showed evidence of considerable

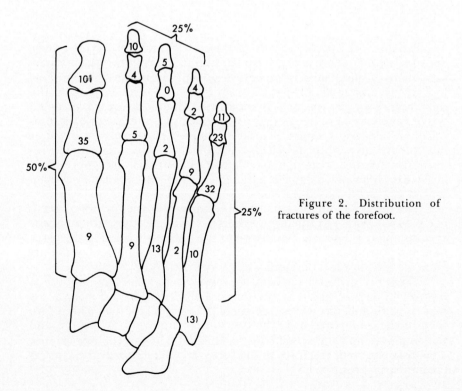

Figure 2. Distribution of fractures of the forefoot.

**Table 1.** *Distribution of 287 Fractures of the Foot in 250 Patients Indicating Average Loss of Working Time\**

| FRACTURES | LARGE TOE RAY | SECOND TOE RAY | THIRD TOE RAY | FOURTH TOE RAY | SMALL TOE RAY |
|---|---|---|---|---|---|
| Third phalanx | — | 10 | 5 | 4 | 11 |
| Second phalanx | 101 (6 out of work an average of 1½ weeks) | 4 | 0 | 2 | 23 |
| First phalanx | 35 (8 out of work an average of 2½ weeks) | 5 (1 out of work for 2 weeks) | 2 | 9 (1 out of work 12 weeks) | 32 (4 out of work an average of 2½ weeks) |
| Metatarsal (43) | 9 (6 out of work an average of 4½ weeks) | 9 (4 out of work an average of 6 weeks; 1 out - 14) | 13 (3 out of work an average of 6 weeks) | 2 | 10 (7 out of work an average of 4½ weeks) |
| Average loss of working time | 2½ weeks | 5 weeks | 6 weeks | 12 weeks | 3½ weeks |
| | 20 patients (50%) | | 9 patients (22.5%) | | 11 patients (27.5%) |

\* Only 40 patients lost over two days of work.

decalcification of all the bones of the foot on the fractured side one year after injury and represented the other case of post traumatic osteoporosis in the series.

Metatarsal fractures were the biggest problem (Table 2). The company series had 43 fractures; two were treated with casts and the remaining patients were treated with semirigid strapping and early ambulation. In the insured group, 15 fractures were all treated with plaster casts or an ambulatory boot cast. There were no open reductions in the insured group and five open reductions in the industrial group. The loss of time in the two groups is also presented in Table 2.

**Table 2.** *Loss of Working Time in Two Series of Patients with Fractures of the Foot*

| | INSURANCE GROUP | INDUSTRIAL GROUP |
|---|---|---|
| Metatarsal fractures | 15 (all with casts) | 43 (two with casts) |
| Time lost | 15 (average time lost was 7½ weeks) | 20 (average time lost was 2 weeks; 14.4 days) (23 lost no time) |
| All fractures | 100 | 250 |
| Time lost | 91 (91%) | 40 (16%) |

**Table 3.**   *Breakdown Cost of All Fractures in 100 Patients from the Insurance Group*

|                                          | TOTAL     | AVERAGE |
|------------------------------------------|-----------|---------|
| Disability days                          | 2,498     | 25      |
| Average weekly wage                      | $12,851   | $128    |
| Wages lost                               | $49,866   | $500    |
| Compensation paid                        | $27,534   | $275    |
| Actual average wage loss (to patient)    |           | $225    |
| Medical paid                             | $ 9,250   | $ 93    |
| Cost to insurer (Compensation and medical) | $36,825 | $368    |

A further study of 100 patients in the insurance group revealed interesting socioeconomic findings as outlined in Table 3. If these studies are further intercalated to 250 patients to compare with the industrial group, the findings are as outlined in Table 4.

## TREATMENT

Initially, fractures of the phalanges are treated with manual positioning of the fracture and loose strapping to a member toe. The patient is then provided with several pairs of fluffy woolen stockings and is fitted with a large oversized work shoe. The shoe is cut out to relieve pressure if necessary (Fig. 3).

If the fracture is more involved and accompanied by a contusion, ice packs are applied initially. An ice-filled vibra-bath appears to discourage hematoma and apparently allows enough local anesthetic effect so that the patient can start early relatively painless ambulation.

Other equipment that has been found to be helpful is a Benson pad. This is a small sponge rubber or lambs' wool cloth-covered packet held with a loop of tubular gauze that is draped over the middle three toes, and renders support to the metatarsal arch. The forefoot can be further stabilized by self-adherent elastic pressure tape, and several layers of fluffy rolled gauze with incorporation of sterilized steel wool between the layers of the gauze. The foot is then compressed and contoured with an elastic bandage; a wooden-soled shoe is applied and immediate ambulation is encouraged (Fig. 4). If necessary, a cane or one crutch is provided so as to encourage weight bearing and immediate ambulation.

**Table 4.**   *Costs of Fractures in the Insurance Group Intercalated to 250 Patients to Compare with the Industrial Group*

|                                | INSURANCE GROUP | INDUSTRIAL GROUP |
|--------------------------------|-----------------|------------------|
| Total lost wages               | $51,000         | $ 9,000          |
| Total compensation medical paid | $83,500        | $15,000          |
| Disability days (all fractures) | 25 days        | 4 days           |

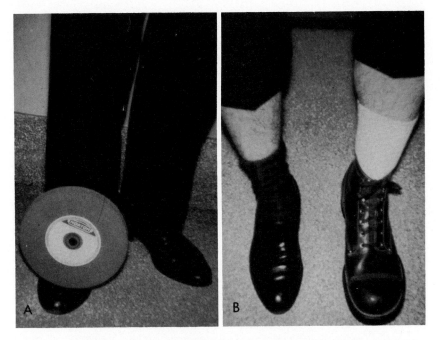

Figure 3. *A*, Direct trauma was the most common mechanism of fractures of the metatarsals and phalanges. *B*, An oversized firm soled work shoe allows comfort and protection to the padded fractured forefoot and allows immediate ambulation.

For fractures of the base of the fifth metatarsal, a half moon shaped piece of adherent felt is applied to the lateral side of the foot and the above routine is instituted. It had been found convenient to use an inexpensive arch support with a semilunar cut-out made at the base of the fifth metatarsal at the point of acute tenderness. A Gibney boot type tape adhesive strapping is then applied to the lower leg to place the foot in slight eversion to relax the pull of the peroneus brevis muscle.

Other convenient adjuncts to the convalescent phase are floor mounted self-service stainless steel foot baths where the patient may soak his feet to remove dressings. These are made with garbage disposal units mounted in the base to dispense the old dressing.

It has been found that treatment with warm soaks or whirlpool foot baths twice daily, when indicated, and the necessary treatment by the industrial nurse once or twice daily is more than repaid by the patient's increased morale and lack of absenteeism.

In the multiply displaced metatarsal, intramedullary fixation is carried out if closed reduction and approximate contact cannot be made. It has been found, however, that the fragments usually mold themselves to the proper level of physiological positioning with correctly applied semirigid support and early ambulation.

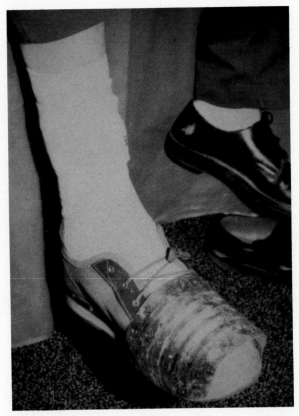

Figure 4.   Commercially wooden-soled shoes, with or without protective steel caps, are useful for immediate ambulation of the padded fractured forefoot.

Recently, the open reduction has been reserved for the completely displaced metatarsal heads. In these, the heaviest Kirschner wire or Steinmann pin that will fit into the proximal intramedullary space is driven proximally.[10] It is cut off at the appropriate level to engage the distal fragments without entering the metatarsophalangeal joint. The usual ambulatory routine is then initiated. There has been no breakage of the internal fixation, no nonunions, and no complication in three such cases. The use of intramedullary Kirschner wire fixation left extruding through the distal skin of the metatarsals is only occasionally used. Its obvious disadvantage is that ambulation cannot be started.

## COMPLICATIONS

The complications have been few. One case of benign thrombophlebitis was thought to be secondary to a fractured metatarsal. Two partial ostectomies have been carried out to relieve painful callus of the forefoot. Two cases of apparent Sudeck's atrophy have been previously mentioned.

Although not a part of this series, similar ambulation has been encouraged with stress or fatigue fractures of the metatarsal. Over the first few months abundant callus is formed, but reabsorption gradually occurs. The apparent force that causes the stress fracture is probably dispelled and the metacarpals adjust themselves to new functional position with subsequent absorption of the redundant callus.

## CONCLUSION

Many fractures of the metatarsals and phalanges have probably been overprotected and overtreated in the past with extreme morbidity and expense to many. Early ambulation expedites bony union and may prevent painful osteoporosis.

Fractures of the forefoot appear to mold themselves to the proper level of physiological positioning with properly applied semirigid support in ambulation. Open reduction of metatarsal fractures is rarely necessary. Angulated and healed fractures of the metatarsals rarely cause functional difficulty. Nonunion of the fracture has not been noted when early ambulation has been effected. A properly applied safety shoe with a protective toe cap would have prevented at least 70 per cent of the fractures presented.

## REFERENCES

1. Benedict, K. T.: Personal communication.

2. Campbell, W.: Personal communication.

3. Cave, E. F. (Editor): Fractures and Other Injuries. Chicago, Year Book Publishers, Inc., 1958.

4. Geckelar, E. O.: Metatarsal resection for disabilities of the foot. Clin. Orthop., 1:187-189, 1949.

5. Giannestras, N. J.: Foot Disorders: Medical and Surgical Management, Philadelphia, Lea & Febiger, 1967.

6. Gissoni, W.: A dangerous type fixation of the foot. J. Bone Joint Surg., 33B:535-538, 1951.

7. Granberry, W. M., and Liscomb, P. L.: Dislocation of the tarsal metatarsal joints. Surg. Gynecol. Obstet., 114:467-469, 1962.

8. Key, J. A., and Conwell, H. E. (Editors): The Management of Fractures, Dislocations, and Sprains. Edition 3. St. Louis, The C. V. Mosby Co., 1942.

9. Lewin, P. (Editor): The Foot and Ankle. Philadelphia, Lea & Febiger, 1940.

10. Lindhold, R.: Operative treatment of the dislocated simple fracture of the neck of the metatarsal bone. Ann. Chir. Gynaec. Fenn., 50:328-331, 1961.

11. McKeever, F. M.: Injuries of the forefoot. American Academy of Orthopedic Surgeons Instructional Course Lectures, Vol. 2, Ann Arbor, J. W. Edwards, 1944.

12. Watson-Jones, R.: Fractures and Joint Injuries. Edition 4. Baltimore, Williams and Wilkins Co., 1955.

## Chapter 21

# Injuries to the Midfoot

### A Major Cause of Industrial Morbidity

RONALD C. HILLEGASS, M.D.*

It has been estimated that of every 300 men working in heavy industry, 15 working days are lost per month as a result of foot problems. Sixty-five per cent of these lost days is a result of trauma. In 1971, it was estimated that over 500 million dollars were paid in compensation in the United States as a result of leg and foot injuries which were work-related.[18]

It is very difficult to obtain good statistics for these injuries in industry. Most state workmen's compensation boards or private insurance carriers categorize a disability under the appropriate anatomic part. There is no effort to separate traumatic from nontraumatic injuries. In an attempt to obtain a lower insurance rate, heavy industry has a strong bias in decreasing the number of accidents involving lost working time. This may result in poor reporting and frequently a man may appear for a full working day although he is unable to do his regular task. Improper diagnosis may also reduce the accuracy of the statistics.

Heavy industry should be complimented on its concern for safety. This may result from financial rather than altruistic motives. Concern with the working environment and education of the worker have resulted in a decreased number of accidents involving lost working time. The enforced use of a safety shoe with a special steel metatarsal protector has also decreased the number of midfoot injuries in industry.

A variety of midfoot injuries are discussed, based on the author's limited experience and the literature is reviewed. Significant injuries to the midfoot are relatively rare, therefore many orthopedic surgeons will be unfamiliar with their diagnosis and treatment. In discussing fractures of the tarsal navicular, Eichenholtz and Levine stated that these injuries were "often neglected, usually unsuspected, frequently undiagnosed, and occasionally mismanaged."[10] This statement is accurate and can

---

* Assistant Surgeon, Department of Orthopedics, Rhode Island Hospital, Providence, Rhode Island.

readily be applied to all injuries of the midfoot; only the use of the word occasionally might be questioned.

The anatomy of the midfoot is well known. It should be emphasized that all bones in the midfoot articulate with at least four bones. The midfoot must function as a stable unit for weight bearing and also must be capable of motion. Anatomists have stated that the lateral border of the foot is functionally specialized as a static, stabilized, supporting organ while the medial aspect of the midfoot is functionally specialized as an elastic, mobile, dynamic organ of propulsion.[15] The plantar ligaments are much stronger than those on the dorsal surface of the foot. Muscle insertions into the midfoot region tend to be on the plantar side of the foot and consequently allow for reinforcement in these areas.[17] The base of the second metatarsal is recessed into the middle cuneiform, resulting in its frequent injury in trauma to the midfoot. In addition there is a strong ligament which goes between the medial cuneiform and the base of the second metatarsal known as Lisfranc's ligament.

Diagnosis of midfoot injuries may be difficult. X-ray examination is essential. Schiller and Ray[19] have outlined criteria to evaluate injuries to the midfoot.

In the normal anteroposterior view of the midfoot, the navicular shadow should overlap all of the cuneiforms equally. In addition there should be no space between the bases of the first and second metatarsals. The sesamoids may provide some clue to the presence or absence of this rotation.

In the lateral view of the foot on x-ray examination, the cuneiforms are noted to overlap and lie directly in line with the navicular; the metatarsals are all superimposed but the shafts should run parallel to each other; and the first metatarsal ray should be the most dorsal. Frequently, comparison views are necessary in evaluating the foot, particularly when trying to determine whether an avulsion fracture exists or that an os tibiale externum is present. Fluoroscopy may provide some help in diagnosing patients in whom there is persistent morbidity involving the midfoot. A subluxation which occurs with motion may be present.

The pathophysiology of injuries to the midfoot has been categorized previously as direct or indirect.[22] Most injuries are probably a combination of these two factors. The direct injuries to the midfoot are self-explanatory and they may be the most dramatic. Primary treatment of severe direct injuries should be directed to obtaining adequate skin coverage and restoring structural stability. Indirect injuries may result from an avulsion secondary to the insertion of a ligament or tendon. The indirect force may also be transmitted to the midfoot as a result of the foot being maintained in a position of plantar flexion.[1] A longitudinal force applied in this fashion will frequently disrupt the weaker dorsal ligamentous structures of the midfoot and result in serious injury. This may be limited to soft tissue injury alone or may be associated with a fracture. Abduction or adduction stress may also cause significant midfoot injuries.

For the purpose of this chapter, midfoot injuries will be discussed as separate entities. However it is imperative to remember that the midfoot is a unit, and that injuries involving one aspect of this unit frequently involve other bones of the midfoot.

## NAVICULAR INJURIES

Fractures of the navicular may be classified as tuberosity, dorsal lip, or body fractures. Avulsion fractures of the tuberosity must be differentiated from an accessory navicular bone. The insertion of the posterior tibial tendon is frequently responsible for these fractures. Usually they respond to immobilization alone; however some authors have advised open reduction and internal fixation if the avulsion fragment is large enough so that the posterior tibial tendon would fail to become functional if the fracture did not heal.[16]

The dorsal lip fracture also responds well to short term immobilization. Cases have been reported in which this dorsal fragment is the major portion of the bone. Again, in these unusual cases, open reduction and internal fixation may be necessary.

Fractures of the body of the navicular may also require open reduction and internal fixation if there is significant displacement of the fracture fragments. Although Watson-Jones[22] devised a technique of skeletal fixation through the os calcis and the base of the metatarsals, more recent authors[10] have advocated reduction and internal fixation with the use of a wire to maintain the reduction.

It is difficult to resolve the problem of severely comminuted fractures of the navicular. Open reduction may be impossible. Watson-Jones and others[10] have advised early arthrodesis of both the talonavicular and the naviculocuneiform joint. It should be noted that this type of treatment is not without problems. In a study of arthrodesis at the naviculocuneiform joint for nontraumatic problems, there were unsatisfactory results in at least 50 per cent at 16 years' follow-up.[20] Severe degenerative changes were present at the talonavicular joint under these conditions.

The high frequency of misdiagnosis in injuries to the navicular is noted in the series of Eichenholtz and Levine.[10] In 67 patients evaluated by them, 17 diagnoses were not made on the initial evaluation. In nine patients, no x-ray films were taken; and in eight additional patients, the diagnosis was not properly identified on evaluation of x-ray films.

## CUBOID INJURIES

Injuries of the cuboid are most frequently avulsion fractures that may be treated with immobilization. Infrequently a more significant fracture involving the body of the cuboid may be present. Cases of dislocation of the cuboid have also been reported.[7] It should be emphasized that the cuboid articulates with five other bones and is crucial for stability on the lateral aspect of the foot. Although Hermel[15] advised early midtarsal fusion for a severe fracture associated with subluxation or dislocation of the cuboid, it is not unreasonable to expect that these injuries would respond well to an accurate reduction and internal fixation if it were possible to perform them. Cases such as those reported by Drummond[7] indicate that good results are possible after an accurate reduction.

## CUNEIFORM INJURY

Cuneiform injury may present a severe problem in diagnosis. Careful evaluation of the x-ray films is essential. Although dislocations of these bones are rare, they do occur as evidenced by a case reported by Schiller and Ray.[19] The correct diagnosis was identified initially. Avulsion fractures may be treated by immobilization. Significant fractures or dislocations must be reduced accurately and internal fixation may be necessary. If a good reduction cannot be achieved, an arthrodesis may be performed. However, the frequency of degenerative changes following this type of fusion must be emphasized.

## TARSOMETATARSAL DISLOCATION

The Lisfranc, or tarsometatarsal dislocation, is a severe injury to the midfoot. Aitken[1] emphasized that this injury may result from either direct or indirect force. With direct force, the metatarsals tend to be dislocated toward the plantar surface. When indirect force causes the dislocation, the metatarsal bases are usually dislocated dorsally. Disruption of the weaker dorsal ligaments occurs. There are frequently fractures of the tarsals and metatarsals in line with the force, especially the second metatarsal or the cuboid. Aitken thought the key to the dislocation to be the base of the second metatarsal, which he believed had to be reduced or resected before reduction could be acccomplished. English[11] stated that the more proximal part of the injury, or the lateral side of the foot, must be reduced to allow the remainder of the foot to be stable. He also thought the interossei muscles contributed significantly to maintain the foot in an unreduced position. Both authors advised an accurate reduction.

The anterior tibial tendon may block closed reduction.[4] If necessary, an open reduction should be performed and internal fixation used when required (Fig. 1). Del Sel[5] described percutaneous pin fixation. Both Aitken[1] and Casselbaum[3] believed that primary fusion between the cuneiforms and metatarsals was rarely indicated.

Although Gissane[12] emphasized the frequency of amputation secondary to disruption of the blood supply as a result of this injury, more recent reports are less pessimistic regarding the incidence of gangrene subsequent to this injury.

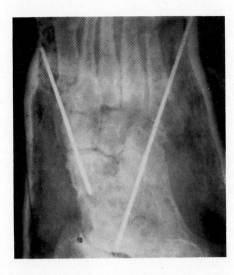

Figure 1. Open reduction of the foot with internal fixation. (*From* Aitken, A. P., and Poulson, D.: Dislocations of the tarsometatarsal joints. J. Bone Joint Surg., 45*A*: 246, 1963, with permission.)

## MIDTARSAL DISLOCATION

Chopart's midtarsal dislocation is an infrequent injury. Watson-Jones stated that this usually resulted from abduction or adduction stress. Stark[21] reported that his dislocation was associated frequently with fractures of the navicular or cuboid. Many of these injuries initially were diagnosed as sprains. Although Watson-Jones felt that closed reduction usually produced good results if there were no associated fractures, Dewar[6] advocated surgical reduction in many of these injuries. Stark emphasized that if the anterior tibial muscle was still intact, conservative treatment should provide a good result. Again accurate reduction appears to be essential. Internal fixation may be necessary. In severe fractures, early midtarsal arthrodesis may be considered.

## SUMMARY

It should be noted that severe injuries to the midfoot are rare. Their infrequent occurrence and the difficulty of diagnosis roentgenographically renders a high level of suspicion essential. All tarsal bones have multiple articular surfaces. Normal functioning of the foot requires pain free motion that tolerates weight bearing. Mild injuries require only immobilization. In more severe injuries, accurate open reduction and internal fixation may be necessary. Although arthrodesis has been favored by a number of authors, it would seem that it should be reserved only for rare instances where comminution is present. Arthrodesis may shorten the early morbidity but increase the long term disability.

# REFERENCES

1. Aitken, A. P., and Poulson, D.: Dislocations of the tarsometatarsal joints. J. Bone Joint Surg., *45A*:246, 1963.

2. Casselbaum, W. H.: Lisfranc fracture-dislocations. Clin. Orthop., *30*:117, 1963.

3. Crenshaw, A. H. (Editor): Campbell's Operative Orthopedics. Edition 5. St. Louis, C. V. Mosby Co., 1971.

4. Collett, H. S., Hood, T. K., and Andrews, R. E.: Tarsometatarsal fracture-dislocations. Surg. Gynecol. Obstet., *106*:623, 1958.

5. Del Sel, J. M.: The surgical treatment of tarso-metatarsal fracture-dislocations. J. Bone Joint Surg., *46B*:700, 1964.

6. Dewar, F. P., and Evans, D. C.: Occult fracture-subluxation of the midtarsal joint. J. Bone Joint Surg., *50B*:386, 1968.

7. Drummond, D. S., and Hastings, D. E.: Total dislocation of the cuboid bone. J. Bone Joint Surg., *51B*:716, 1969.

8. Easton, E. R.: Two rare dislocations of the metatarsals at Lisfranc's joint. J. Bone Joint Surg., *20*:1053, 1938.

9. Eftekhar, N. M., Lyddon, D. W., and Stevens, J.: An unusual fracture-dislocation of the tarsal navicular. J. Bone Joint Surg., *51B*:716, 1969.

10. Eichenholtz, S. N., and Levine, D. B.: Fractures of the tarsal navicular bone. Clin. Orthop., *34*:142, 1964.

11. English, T. A.: Dislocations of the metatarsal bone and adjacent toe. J. Bone Joint Surg., *46B*:700, 1964.

12. Gissane, W.: A dangerous type of fracture of the foot. J. Bone Joint Surg., *33B*:535, 1951.

13. Granberry, W., and Lipscomb, P. B.: Dislocation of the tarsometatarsal joints. Surg. Gynecol. Obstet., *114*:467, 1962.

14. Heck, C. V.: Fractures of the bones of the foot (except the talus). Surg. Clin. North Amer., *45*:103, 1965.

15. Hermel, M. B., and Gershon-Cohen, J.: The nutcracker fracture of the cuboid by indirect violence. Radiology, *60*:850, 1953.

16. Holstein, A., and Joldersma, R. D.: Dislocation of first cuneiform in tarsometatarsal fracture-dislocation. J. Bone Joint Surg., *32A*:419, 1950.

17. Jeffreys, T. E.: Lisfranc's fracture-dislocation. J. Bone Joint Surg., *45B*:546, 1963.

18. National Safety Council: Accident facts, 1971.

19. Schiller, M. G., and Ray, R. D.: Isolated dislocation of the medial cuneiform bone A rare injury of the tarsus. J. Bone Joint Surg., *52A*:1632, 1970.

20. Seymour, N.: The late results of naviculo-cuneiform fusion. J. Bone Joint Surg., *49B*:558, 1967.

21. Stark, W.: Occult fracture-subluxation of the mid-tarsal joint. Clin. Orthop., *93*:291, 1973.

22. Watson-Jones, R.: Fractures and Joint Injuries. Edition 4. Baltimore, Williams and Wilkins Co., 1960.

23. Wiley, J. J.: The mechanism of tarso-metatarsal joint injuries. J. Bone Joint Surg., *53B*:474, 1971.

24. Wilson, P. D.: Fractures and dislocations of the tarsal bones. Southern Med. J., *26*:833, 1933.

*Chapter 22*

# Safety Shoes for Industry

NATHANIEL GOULD, M.D.*

The foot is the most vulnerable part of the body subjected to injury in industry. The total national work force is roughly estimated at 85 million and, of course, includes the military forces of the United States.

For many years, there have been standards of development in the manufacture of shoes both with regard to materials and performance, propounded by the War Production Board. In 1940, a program for the development of safety shoes for all industry was begun and originally was based on the American War Standards. The National Safety Council and the American Insurance Association took on the development of this project. The committee which evolved was labeled the Z-41 Committee. In 1962, an approved membership was reviewed and established. The first meeting was held in 1963. Subcommittees were also organized and standards for this Z-41 series, based on the American War Standards, were reviewed, revised, and brought up to date as special requirements for various industries evolved.

## THE NATIONAL SAFETY COUNCIL

In 1912, a small group "concerned with industrial safety" met in Chicago and discussed the organization of a "council" which would be a "nonprofit, nongovernmental, public service organization dedicated to safety education and the development of accident prevention programs."

On September 24, 1913, The National Council for Industrial Safety was formed, the name changed the following year to the National Safety Council. A charter was granted by the United States Congress on August 13, 1953, "to arouse and maintain the interest . . . in safety and in accident prevention, and to encourage the adoption and institution of safety methods by all persons, corporations and other organizations." Headquarters for this self-governing, self-disciplining organization remains

---

* Chief of Orthopedic Service, Brockton Hospital, Brockton, Massachusetts; Senior Orthopedic Surgeon, Massachusetts Hospital School, Canton, Massachusetts.

in Chicago. Its membership is composed of "more than 15,000 individuals and organizations including manufacturers, transportation carriers, insurance companies, public utilities, hospitals, governmental agencies, associations, schools and all manner of citizen service groups." Its Board of Trustees are volunteers from the membership. There is a "continuous flow of information on safety, to and from the membership." Unfortunately, not all of the components of industry associate themselves with the safety movement and only 25 to 30 per cent of the national work force is involved. Finances come from membership dues and from various materials and services performed under contract. Similar safety programs exist in other countries.

## Z-41 COMMITTEE

The following organizations were in the original listing of the Z-41 Committee:

1. American Federation of Labor and Congress of Industrial Organization
2. American Gas Association
3. American Insurance Association
4. American Iron and Steel Institute
5. American Metal Stamping Association
6. American Mining Congress
7. American Mutual Insurance Alliance
8. American Petroleum Institute
9. American Society of Safety Engineers
10. Associated General Contractors of America
11. Association of American Railroads
12. Electric Light and Power Group
13. Holland-Racine Shoes, Incorporated
14. Industrial Safety Equipment Association
15. International Association of Government Labor Officials
16. International Shoe Company
17. Iron Age Safety Shoe Company
18. Lehigh Safety Shoe Company
19. Manufacturing Chemists Association
20. J. F. McElwain Company
21. National Association of Shoe Chain Stores
22. National Footwear Manufacturers Association, Incorporated
23. National Safety Council
24. Record Industrial Company
25. Safety Box Toe Company
26. Safety First Shoe Company
27. Telephone Group
28. Thom McAn Shoe Company
29. Underwriters Laboratories, Incorporated
30. United States Department of Agriculture
31. United States Department of the Army
32. United States Department of the Interior, Bureau of Mines
33. United States Department of the Navy, Office of Industrial Relations

Several years ago, the American Academy of Orthopaedic Surgeons was added. During this past year, the 1967 standards were reviewed and revised. The standards provide specifications, performance requirements, and methods of testing for safety footwear designed primarily to protect the feet of the wearer.

Specifications have been instituted for protection of the toes, the metatarsal regions, penetration of the shoe from below, electrical conduction, and for protection from electrical hazards. No attempt is made to specify the exact materials since it is felt that plastics, for example, may suddenly appear that would satisfy the requirements and if specific materials were specified, it would be necessary to revise all the listed specifications and would cause a constant upheaval in the development and manufacture of such safety shoes. The armed forces, however, have reserved the right to specify materials to be used.

By following the precepts as outlined by the committee, injuries have been reduced by more than 70 per cent.

## SAFETY TOES

Safety footwear material is simply listed as being suitably constructed for the exposure it is intended to receive and should provide comfort and wearability and comply with the standards of the compression and impact testing necessary for its listed role. A protective toe box is employed that is incorporated into the footwear during construction and becomes part of the footwear.

### Impact Testing

Unworn size 9 D men's footwear is selected at random from stock and three specimens from each style are employed. At least 14 days must have elapsed since the completion of their manufacture. The test specimen is then cut out and placed in position under the impact testing apparatus (Fig. 1). The impact testing equipment (Fig. 2) is a weight of steel

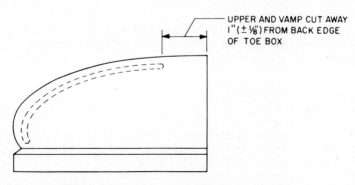

UPPER AND VAMP CUT AWAY
1" ($\pm$ ⅛") FROM BACK EDGE
OF TOE BOX

Figure 1.   Toe box prepared for impact testing.

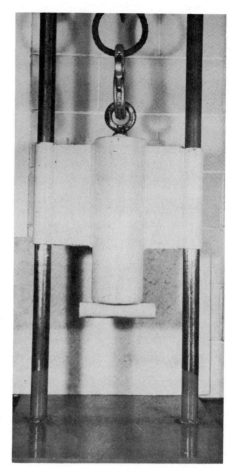

Figure 2. Machine for impact testing.

which falls freely from the vertical height with the plunger one inch in diameter and six inches long. The bottom striking surface of the plunger is rounded to a one inch radius. The upper end of the plunger has a two inch diameter, a ¼ inch thick steel plate screwed to it, which is replaced if at any time it is found to be worn or damaged. The base on which the testing equipment is supported is usually constructed of steel and has a mass of not less than 500 pounds since it is necessary to minimize the absorption of energy which might adversely affect test results. The point of the impact of the plunger strikes in the approximate center of the toe box about ½ inch in front of its back edge.

The proper class footwear, measured in foot pounds, is determined by the weight of the material dropped plus the height from which it falls. Therefore footwear has been classified as 75 footwear (50 pound weight from the height of 18 inches), 50 footwear (50 pound weight from the height of 12 inches), and 30 footwear (50 pound weight from the height of 7¼ inches). The owner of the factory or industry where the worker is to wear the safety shoe determines just how well the foot of his worker should be protected, judging by the possible weight of material falling in his particular environment. The strength of the supporting material at the point of impact should not reduce the inside vertical height of the toe box of the shoe to less than ½ inch.

Measurement of a number of great toes of patients showed that the vertical height of the average adult great toe was about one inch, so that one could assume that there might be some crush of soft tissue by the impact but probably elimination of fracture. Shoes for an appropriate industry should exceed test requirements expected from a maximal impact.

## Compression Testing

The same cutout specimens of footwear utilized for impact testing are also used for compression testing (Fig. 3). The testing machine (Fig. 4) is equipped with compression testing surfaces that remain parallel during loads of up to 5000 pounds. Compression test shoes must pass a loading of 1000 to 5000 pounds plus or minus a 50 pound variable and are so listed in their classification. Here again the owner of the plant selects the shoe which he feels is necessary for any compression accidents which may occur in his particular plant. Since compression testing may, in different hands, result in so many variables with many variations of reports, and is also expensive to be carried out, this type of testing has been given up by practically all foreign countries. In the United States, since nearly all injuries arise from impact and because of the uncertainty and variability in compression testing, here too this type of testing of footwear will probably be eliminated in the near future. Up to the present, it has provided a check and balance method to insure that a proper, sturdy sole material be incorporated in the manufacture of safety shoes. The armed forces, where the exact ingredients of sole materials are specified, have given up on compression testing.

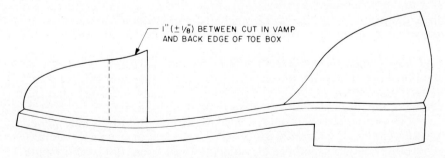

1″(± ⅛″) BETWEEN CUT IN VAMP
AND BACK EDGE OF TOE BOX

Figure 3.   Footwear with vamp and upper cut away facilitate compression testing.

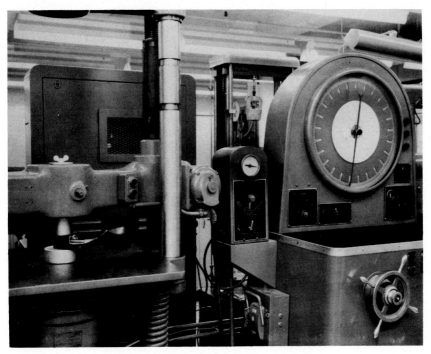

Figure 4.   Machine for compression testing.

## METATARSAL FOOTWEAR

Test footwear consists of a size 9 D shoe with a wax form inserted into the test shoe. The wax form is prepared in specific fashion with specific materials, largely of paraffin and bees wax in a proportion of five to one, then heated and mixed in such a way as to eliminate all bubbles and to obtain a uniformity of material. The testing is done at approximately room temperature. The impact testing equipment is as for the safety toe shoes but the point of impact of the test weight is $3\frac{3}{8}$ inches back from the forward tip of the toe, following a line centered between the heel and the toe axis (Fig. 5). A class 75 metatarsal safety footwear has a clearance before testing of $1\frac{1}{2}$ inches and after impact of one inch. The average metatarsal region in men's feet was $1\frac{7}{8}$ inches which would suggest that there would be some soft tissue crush at this point of impact but probably no fracture. However because of a bulkiness and lack of cosmetics in the manufacture of footwear that would provide 100 per cent protection in this category, no changes were made in the test requirements. Owners of plants were encouraged to purchase footwear that would survive a test somewhat higher than what would be felt to be necessary to prevent impact injuries in that plant. Figure 6 shows cutout shoes which have incorporated various safety features.

## MEN'S CONDUCTIVE SHOES

These shoes are intended to provide protection from static electricity that may accumulate on personnel and are designed to dissipate this static electricity to the ground and prevent the ignition of sensitive explosive mixtures. They are also intended for use by personnel operating high voltage lines when the potential on the person and the energized part must be equal. The footwear intended to dissipate static electricity has been designated as Type I and that for high voltage linesmen, Type II. It is important in this type of footwear that all exposed external metal parts be nonferrous. Type I footwear requires a nonmetallic heel. Zinc is commonly used for the nonferrous metal. The nailheads are below the tread surface, so-called blind nailing.

Type I footwear has an electrical resistance in new or unworn shoes ranging between 25,000 and 500,000 ohms. Type II footwear has an electrical resistance involving each conductive component and sock lining not exceeding 10,000 ohms when measured. I shall not go into the intricacies of electrical measurement except to state that this is done with a suitably calibrated ohmmeter.

After the shoe passes the proper testing, it is identified by a three-lined stamp: the first line representing the American National Standards Institute (ANSI); the second line indicating the type of shoe, in this case, conductive shoe and the Type (I or II); and the third line, Z-41.3-1973/30. The third line represents the ANSI standard number and date of approval with the number following the slash mark indicating test results for impact and compression as required.

Floor oils, oily cleaning compounds, or some particular floor waxes cannot be used on floors where conductive shoes are to be worn. The shoes themselves, in order to function properly, particularly with the soles and the heels, should be clean at all times. Grit and corrosion products and oils damage the effectiveness of conductive shoes. Because wool has an insulating property, the wearers of these shoes connot wear woolen stockings but must wear slightly dampened but clean cotton, rayon, or nylon materials. Foot powders tend to insulate and dry and

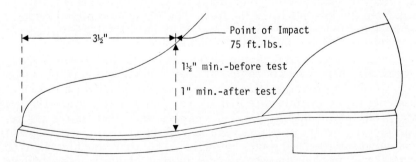

Figure 5.   Method of impact testing (metatarsal).

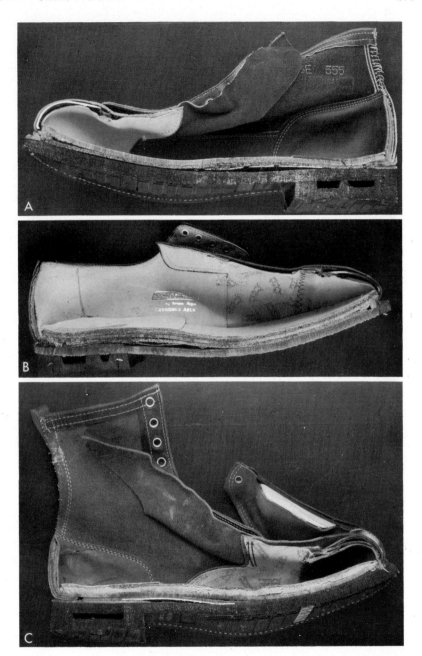

Figure 6. *A*, Men's short all-purpose boot, soft leather, lined for comfort. Other features include steel safety toe, steel heel protector, and steel shank. The thick neoprene sole and heel are nonskid and difficult to penetrate. *B*, Men's dress oxford with cushioned arch, steel safety toe, steel shank, thick sole, and Goodyear welt. *C*, Men's high top, soft leather boot with cushioned arch, steel safety toe, steel shank, protective leather reinforced tongue, stiffened reinforced leather heel protection, and thick, nonskid, highly impentrable neoprene sole and heel.

also should not be used. A conductive sock lining should not be removed from the shoes nor should it be separated because this may create excessively high resistance or may show up as a break in the circuit. These shoes should be tested periodically, Type I shoes being withdrawn from use when the electrical resistance exceeds one million ohms and Type II when the electrical resistance exceeds 10,000 ohms.

## ELECTRICAL HAZARD SHOES

These shoes are intended to provide protection against open circuits of less than 600 volts under dry conditions and are not intended to supplant conditions where conductive footwear is required. They protect the toes from an impact force. The shoes also must have safety toe boxes incorporated during their construction. No metal parts may be present in the sole or heel of the shoe. The outsole of the shoe is a highly electrically resistant composition not less than 12 irons (one iron equals 1/40 of an inch) in thickness. The heels are whole heels of electrically resistant composition.

Three sample shoes, new and unworn, about 14 days from date of manufacture, are tested in a dry, nondestructive environment. The inside of the shoe is covered with a sufficient amount of distilled water to cover the insole for about five minutes and then the water is poured out and the shoe tested immediately for current leakage. The exact type of transformer specified should be used. The shoe is also tested utilizing a five pound weighted foil electrode placed within the shoe in contact with at least 60 per cent of the surface of the insole.

If the shoe passes the test, then it is identified as previously stated for conductive shoes, except "electrical hazard shoe" is listed on the second line. Periodically worn electrical hazard shoes are tested to ascertain whether the insulating properties of the footwear remain.

## WOMEN'S SAFETY SHOES

Specifications for women's safety shoes have not as yet been fully propounded. At present, in situations where a woman is doing the work that ordinarily, in the past, has been relegated to a man, she is expected to wear the same type of safety shoes that men wear. However it is often more difficult to enforce the wearing of safety shoes with women than it is with men because of the lack of elegant, cosmetic appearance of some of the specifically required footwear. With the advent of more women in industry, safety shoe regulations specifically outlined for women with slightly different requirements, will have to be considered.

## SPORTS

There is, at present, much experimental work going on with regard to safety precautions in footwear for various sports. One reads frequently about the increase in injuries to the lower extremities with the advent of artificial turf. With the variations in types of artificial turf, one finds that requirements for cleats, and so forth, on footwear necessarily differ in order to eliminate, as much as possible, injuries to the lower extremities. There is a marked variable here as compared with requirements for grass conditions. With the intense investigations underway, it may be expected that some time within the not too distant future, adequate safety footwear will evolve.

Much work has been done in the manufacture of proper footwear for ski enthusiasts and ice skaters. However, with the improvement in this footwear and better stabilization of the foot and the ankle, there has been an increase in leg and knee injuries. These problems must also be solved.

## MILITARY FOOTWEAR

Even though the thought or mention of war is abhorrent to most individuals, if and when circumstances do lead to such a conflict, it behooves us to protect our fighting forces from the injuries and illnesses germane to their environment by providing them with proper and adequate equipment. Improper footwear can affect the combat efficiency of any force and careful development of proper materials is constantly made and reviewed.

### Navy

A review of Naval casualties during the era of World War II revealed that footwear used on decks of ships soaked up water and rapidly deteriorated. The all leather footwear had originally been designed for land wear and the constancy of wet feet resulted in numerous incapacities. It was noted that the upper leather would split after constant wetting and recurring drying and that insoles, which were vegetable tanned, cracked after short periods of wear.

The decks of a ship are constantly splashed with water and it was necessary to discover footwear which could be protected from the "corrosive elements of the sea." The new water resistant Fleet shoe is made of water resistant leather, has nonmarking heels and soles, and polyethylene counters. The shoe seams are so constructed that they bar penetration of water through the stitch holes. This has now become the "general purpose shoe, the field shoe, the flight deck shoe" and eliminates the need for wearing rubbers with work shoes. This is now the work shoe of the Fleet instead of the previous three different types of work shoes. This shoe has proven itself effective in barring penetration of water. Its components are sufficiently durable and suitable so that they may be used on both wet and dry terrain. They are inexpensive. Further investigation is being carried out, particularly with regard to vulcanization construction.

## Army

Booby traps of "Panji" spikes were prevalent throughout Southeast Asia in the combat of the past number of years. A tropical combat boot was designed, and insoles of stainless steel plates .012 of an inch thick were employed and were effective in resisting penetration from these spikes. There are also boots designed for the temperate zone and for Arctic and Antarctic usage. Light weight comfort shoes are made with an open weave material resulting in high air permeability for personnel on rest and recuperation leave.

A tropical combat boot was designed which frees itself fairly readily of mud and maintains a relatively consistent traction capability. The outsole design was developed during the Vietnam War.

A standardized dress shoe is now employed for all four services. Various measurements were taken of over 20,000 soldiers and a comfortable shoe came into being. It was similar to the old Munson last designed during the period of World War I and has a straight inside last and wide outflare for the toes. The toe box is sufficiently deep to allow enough room for the toes.

For the sake of economy and ease of delivery, research is being carried out and will continue to be carried out for material which will be proper to insert into a combat boot to render it all purpose or suitable to be worn in the Arctic with temperatures as low as $-20$ degrees F. or in the warm climates with temperatures as high as 100 degrees F.

## SUMMARY

Statistics have shown that the foot is a most vulnerable part of the body and liable to injury in almost every industry. This applies equally in both military and civilian endeavors.

With these factors in mind and aided by the longstanding know-how of the military, standards for design and manufacture have been propounded through a committee labeled Z-41 of the National Safety Council, with membership composed of approximately 30 representatives, manufacturers, and utilizers of safety shoes for industry and the armed forces. The parent National Safety Council, a self-developing, self-governing, and self-disciplining body, is a voluntary effort of American industry to protect its manpower work force and to eliminate any elements which could impair the industrial economy of the nation.

Methods of testing safety toe and safety metatarsal footwear are outlined and basic requirements for electrical hazard and conductive shoes and other varied safety features are provided. Up-to-date military footwear is reviewed.

People are people, and unfortunately are sometimes careless about self-protection and still suffer injury to themselves with subsequent loss of income simply by forgetting to utilize the safeguards that have been provided for them. Emergency rooms of hospitals are beset with injuries which could have been lessened or easily eliminated if the injured party had not carelessly omitted the use of such safety footwear. It is hoped that labor unions, by making definitive demands upon their membership, will require that the labor force utilize the safety measures that have been provided for them.

American industry has made rapid strides in these safety endeavors and better and better materials are constantly being discovered and exploited.

ACKNOWLEDGMENTS

The author wishes to acknowledge the assistance of the following persons in preparation of this paper: Paul Sheppard, Secretary, National Safety Council; A. J. Ferrara, Staff Engineer, U. S. Steel Corporation, Monroeville, Pennsylvania; Harvey Childs, Jr., Vice-President, Iron Age Shoe Co., Pittsburgh, Pennsylvania; Milton Bailey and Douglas Swain, Natick Laboratories, United States Army, Natick Massachusetts; and fellow members of the Z-41 Committee.

## REFERENCES

1. National Safety Council: Booklet on Development and Aims. Chicago.
2. National Safety Council: U.S.A. Standards, Z-41 Committee. Chicago.

*Chapter 23*

# Injuries of the Foot
# in Dancers

WILLIAM A. LIEBLER, M.D.*

Under the heading of industrial injuries of the foot and ankle, injuries of the foot in dancers may be included. My experience in this area began when I first became interested in ballet dancers in 1956 under the eye of the late Henry Jordan, whose understanding and work with dancers was phenomenal.

Basic motions of ballet must be understood by the practicing physician so that he can intelligently treat conditions of the foot.

Whereas the average dancer starts training at approximately five years of age and may continue dancing until the age of 40 or rarely 60; the youngest dancer in this series was 13 years of age and the oldest was 48 years of age. Thirty per cent of the 1000 ballet injuries were covered by the workmen's compensation benefits. Of these, there was a ratio of six women to one man, with the number of men participating in dancing slowly increasing over the years. Also, the number of dancers now covered by workmen's compensation appears to be increasing.

It is hard to isolate the foot as the only area sustaining injuries, as most dancers' injuries entail not only the foot, but the ankle, the leg, and many times, the knee. The usual ingrown toenails and soft corns are rarely seen by the the orthopedic surgeon. One has to remember that in the majority of cases the ballet dancer usually has been seen by a podiatrist, chiropodist, masseuse, dance therapist, physiotherapist, chiropractor, osteopath, and it seems when all else fails, the dancer consults an orthopedic surgeon.

Twenty-six per cent of the injuries in this group were ankle sprains. Sprains and strains of dancers are no different from those of other patients and their treatment is usually the same, with the exception of the desire for the least amount of immobilization so that dancing may be resumed as soon as possible. Most sprains usually involve the anterolateral ligaments rather than the posterior or inferior ligaments. On the medial aspect, the posterior and anterior aspects of the medial collateral ligament appear to be equally involved. Approximately 4 per cent of the sprains

---

* Attending, Lenox Hill Hospital, New York, New York; Consultant to American Ballet Theater, New York City Ballet, Robert Joffrey, Agnes De Mille, Martha Graham, Alvin Ailey City Dance Co.; Team Physician, New York Rangers.

involve the forefoot, 4 per cent the metatarsophalangeal joints, and 2 per cent the interphalangeal joints. The majority of all sprains have concomitant tendinitis, or tenosynovitis, or both, with involvement of the ankle in 13 per cent and the foot in 5 per cent. With mild sprains, dancers are usually able to work within a week, moderate sprains in about three weeks, and severe sprains, especially when the ligaments are torn, in about three months.

Tendinitis and tenosynovitis appear to be common afflictions of the foot and ankle in dancers. The occasional use of cortisone injections into the affected area may be effective, but successful results have been achieved by rest, phenylbutazone, and strapping. Overall, whether the tendinitis is in a dancer, a football player, or hockey player, rest appears to be the most important factor.

In chronic tendinitis, when all else fails, radiation therapy to the involved area may be useful, in fractionated doses of approximately 800 roentgens. When the tendinitis is severe, plaster immobilization is effected with a walking plaster boot and radiation through the plaster.

Morton's neuroma, classically occurring between the third and fourth interspaces, was seen in approximately 4 per cent of the cases in this series. True metatarsalgia was seen in less than 1 per cent of the cases. Symptomatic hallux valgus and hallux rigidus were evident occasionally. Surgical procedures for correction of this condition is rarely indicated if the dancer desires to continue ballet.

Arthritis is usually seen most frequently in the first metatarsophalangeal joint and may be treated with phenylbutazone or other anti-inflammatory agents, in addition to modified supports such as dancers' pads.

Two per cent of the dancers had sesamoiditis, which may cripple a dancer. This condition responds to phenylbutazone or injection of a small amount of cortisone into the most painful area. Occasionally the sesamoid may have to be removed.

The incidence of accessory navicula was 1 per cent in this series. The dancer is usually not aware of the condition until a forceful strain is put upon this area, most commonly by developing a new technique, dancing on a surface that is too hard, or overwork. The occurrence of accessory naviculas was usually unilateral; however approximately five were bilateral. One accessory navicula was excised, and at present another may require excision.

Freiberg's necrosis occurred in 1.2 per cent of the dancers. A 14 year old dancer experienced pain and tenderness in the forefoot; subsequent x-ray films revealed development of Freiberg's necrosis in its initial stages. The forefoot healed after a year of rest and the patient was able to resume dancing.

One young patient with the same condition did not desire to rest but elected to continue dancing. A year later she began to experience pain and developed a permanent deformity of the metatarsal heads that is still symptomatic.

Fractures constitute 13 per cent of the injuries sustained by dancers.

The base of the fifth metatarsal appears to be a common area of fracture. Nonunion of this fracture, which is relatively rare, occurred in one patient. The foot remained mildly symptomatic but the patient did not desire surgery and continued dancing. An overworked, overtired dancer may hear something snap in the foot when coming down from a leap. X-ray films usually reveal a fracture of the fifth metatarsal. The fracture usually heals within eight to 12 weeks and dancing may be resumed. One patient started dancing too soon after sustaining this type of fracture and while placing her weight on her opposite foot, suddenly twisted it, breaking the proximal phalanx of the second and third toes, causing a loss of eight additional weeks before she could return to dancing.

The dancer's foot is sensitive to floor surfaces. I have seen several patients who have danced outdoors during the summer on hard terrazzo surfaces, only to develop pain, especially in the dorsum of the feet. Two patients developed pain and tenderness in the dorsum of the feet and both had small undisplaced fractures at the base of the second metatarsals. Hypertrophy of the second metatarsal is a common finding usually resulting from prolonged dancing.

Another patient in this series, a girl 18 years of age, sustained a hyperflexion injury to the metatarsophalangeal joint. X-ray films revealed displacement of half of the head of the second metatarsal, and fracture of the medial condyle of the proximal phalanx of the third toe. Open reduction was carried out and replacement of the displaced bony fragment was anatomically fixed with two Kirschner wires in a cross pin manner. Six weeks later the pins were removed and healing was complete. Three months later she resumed dancing lessons and six months later was able to ballet.

Pain in the ankle may often be caused by a fracture that has not been diagnosed. In one instance a patient experienced pain in his ankle after completing a jump. Because of persistent pain and tenderness, x-ray films were taken revealing a minimally displaced fracture of the medial malleolus. After six weeks of immobilization and an additional six weeks of reconditioning, the patient was able to dance again.

Small chips, which may represent chip fractures of the tip of the malleoli, both in the medial and lateral aspects of the ankle, are common and usually are residual evidence of inversion-eversion types of sprains.

Fractures of the sesamoid bones occurred in two patients in this series. Radiographically, they are often difficult to visualize, and should be treated on a clinical basis. In dancers, the medial sesamoid bone seems to be the only one to sustain fractures.

An interesting phenomenon one sees as a vocational hazard is impingement exostosis in the tibial talar articulation. A lateral x-ray view taken of the foot in flexion and in extension is invaluable in exposing the site of impingement and the mechanism thereof. Bilateral symptomatic exostosis may be an indication for surgery.

Arthritic changes in the fibular talar mortise may be seen in conjunction with the impingement syndrome. This condition was present bilaterally in one patient and surgery was necessary to relieve discomfort. Impingement exostosis of the first metatarsophalangeal joint is also seen occasionally. Surgery is indicated when there is no response to symptomatic treatment.

## CONCLUSION

In regard to all injuries in dancers, whether compensable or not, the dancer's only desire is to resume dancing as soon as possible. It is encumbent upon the orthopedist, insofar as possible, to assist in the accomplishment of this goal. From a compensable point of view, it is difficult to explain to the insuring company or at compensation hearings that when treating a dancer, routine guidelines are not appropriate. Not only must the injury heal, but a substantial amount of time must be spent reconditioning the injured foot and the associated muscles and ligaments in order to regain muscle tone and strength and flexibility and balance.

# Index

289